Reviews

"The physician and writer John Geyman has delivered again an updated portrait of American medical care in 2019. His new book describes the controversies clearly, dissects the myths that are growing like weeds as universal health insurance rises to the top of the political agenda, and makes plain why the remedies of increasing competition among insurance giants will surely not produce the health care Americans want and increasingly do not get. Geyman is the Consumer Report[er] of our medical policy debates. He clearly provides a portrait of where American medicine is as we face the presidential race of 2020."

—Theodore Marmor, Ph.D., professor emeritus of public policy and management at Yale University, author of *The Politics of Medicare* (2013), and member of the National Academy of Medicine

"A bizarre twist of American exceptionalism is that we have by far the most expensive health care system in the world, and yet it is one of the poorest performing of well financed systems. Particularly egregious are the poor health outcomes of not only many of those who remain uninsured but also of the tens of millions who are insured but their coverage fails them in time of medical need. John Geyman explains what is wrong, what the political failures are that led to this fiasco, and, most importantly, what we can do to finally bring us a high performance system that is affordable and accessible for each and everyone of us."

—Don McCanne, M.D., family physician, senior health policy fellow and past president of Physicians for a National Health Program (PNHP)

"Dr. John Geyman has done more than anyone I know to not only explain just how unfair and dysfunctional the American health care system has become but to also show us the way forward. His latest book details the consequences of an administration hell bent on aiding health insurers and other profiteers at the expense of the rest of us. Just as important, it lays out the steps we as a country must take and explains why incremental change won't work. "

—Wendell Potter, Founder of Tarbell, Author of *Deadly Spin* and *Nation on the Take*

Dr. Geyman's Annual Exam...

"Like any good personal physician, Dr. John Geyman has once again performed his complete annual examination and reported on our most concerning patient: the ailing U.S. Health Care System. The news isn't good. In fact, it's a lot worse: "Struggling and Dying Under Trumpcare". Geyman's updated facts and analysis are as clear and reliable as ever. More Americans (29 million) are uninsured, and still more (85 million) are underinsured. In the wake of Trump's failure to repeal Obamacare, it remains an emasculated system bereft of the many benefits it provided, such as protection from denial for pre-existing conditions. With no legitimate replacement, private health insurance and pharmaceutical costs are more firmly than ever in the hands of the profiteers, while Americans die, go bankrupt or both, increasingly unable to access affordable health services.

The good news, Geyman argues, is there is an affordable cure. In a true, traditional Medicare for All—through savings of private insurer costs, negotiated drug prices, bulk purchasing and a fair progressive tax—95% of Americans would pay less than they do now for all their insurance and healthcare. It would cover everyone. Dr. Geyman shows us the way."

—Rick Flinders, M.D., family physician and former long-term
educator at the Santa Rosa Family Medicine Residency,
Sutter Santa Rosa Regional Hospital, Santa Rosa, CA

"Americans are suffering from the Trump administration rolling back benefits while drug prices and premiums have risen astronomically. The medical industrial complex is thriving while the average consumer suffers from poor access, low quality and inflated prices. The private health insurance system is not serving us well and becoming unaffordable for families. Dr. Geyman shows the way forward in this important book. We can have better health care access, higher quality and more affordable insurance if we follow rational economic policies already in place in the rest of the developed world. Americans deserve better: a single payer improved Medicare for All."

—Charles Q. North, M.D., MS, Indian Health Service Chief Medical
Officer, retired Captain USPHS, professor of family and
community medicine, University of New Mexico

STRUGGLING AND DYING UNDER TRUMPCARE

How We Can Fix This Fiasco

John Geyman, M.D.

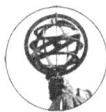

Copernicus Healthcare
Friday Harbor, WA

Struggling and Dying Under Trumpcare
How We can Fix This Fiasco

John Geyman, M.D.

Copernicus Healthcare
Friday Harbor, WA

Ingram Edition
Copyright ©2019 by John Geyman, M.D. All rights reserved

Book design, cover and illustrations by W. Bruce Conway
Cover image used under license from Shutterstock.com
Author photo by Anne Sheridan

softcover: ISBN: 978-1-938218-24-8

Library of Congress Control Number: 2019938946

Copernicus Healthcare
34 Oak Hill Drive
Friday Harbor, WA 98250

www.copernicus-healthcare.org

Dedication

To all Americans who deserve universal coverage for health care with full access at an affordable cost, and with quality that our system can provide. May you see reform, through your activism, that provides assurance to this care based on medical necessity and returns American medicine to its traditional ethic of service.

CONTENTS

Tables and Figures

ACKNOWLEDGMENTS

As with my previous books, I am indebted to many for making this book possible. Thanks are due to many investigative journalists, health professionals, and others for their probing reports on our increasingly dysfunctional health care system. The work of many organizations has been helpful in gathering evidence-based information on what is actually happening at both a macro and micro level as it impacts patients and their families. I have found reports from the Kaiser Family Foundation and its Kaiser Health News especially helpful, together with Dr. Don McCanne's Quote of the Day (don@mccanne.org) that draws widely from so many sources. Reports from other organizations that have also been helpful include the Center for National Health Program Studies, the Centers for Medicare and Medicaid Services, the Commonwealth Fund, the Congressional Budget Office, the Office of Inspector General, the Organization for Economic Cooperation and Development, Public Citizen's Health Research Group, the U. S. Government Accountability Office, and the World Health Organization.

W. Bruce Conway, my colleague at Copernicus Healthcare over many years, has once again done a great job from start to finish of this book, including cover design, interior layout, and conversion to e-book format. Carolyn Acheson has created a useful, reader-friendly index.

Many thanks to my ten colleagues who read advance copies of the book and contributed their generous comments as brief reviews. Most of all, I am grateful to my wife, Emily, for her careful reading and suggestions through many drafts, including editing, proofing, and promotion of the final book.

PREFACE

The 2018 mid-term elections were a watershed moment in American politics. After the highest off-year voter turnout in a mid-term election in 50 years, Democrats won the national congressional vote by a margin greater than that of the Tea Party Republicans in 2010 and women turned farther away from the Republican Party. Democrats retook the House and gained seats in the Republican-controlled Senate. There are now progressive Democratic presidential candidates, and more than 40 new Democratic members bring increased progressive energy to the House. The new Congressional Progressive Caucus is projected to include about 40 percent of House Democrats. What to do about our dysfunctional and cruel health care system, made worse over the first two years of the Trump administration, was a leading domestic issue in the mid-terms, as it will be for the 2020 campaigns.

As has been true for years, the ultimate goal of the progressive wing of the Democratic Party remains to enact universal coverage for all Americans through Expanded and Improved Medicare for All. Since 2003, it has been in the House as H. R. 676, sponsored by Rep. John Conyers (Dem. MI). A new, updated bill has been introduced by Rep. Pramila Jayapal (Dem. WA) as H. R. 1384, the Medicare for All Act of 2019, already with 107 co-sponsors. House Speaker Nancy Pelosi has agreed to have hearings on the bill, which are expected to be held in several committees. On the Senate side, Senator Bernie Sanders remains the lead sponsor for a similar bill as S-1804, with 14 co-sponsors.

As has been true in previous years, a coalition of corporate stakeholders, led especially by Big PhRMA and America's Health Insurance Plans (AHIP), the trade organization of private health insurers, and allied interests are organizing to oppose Medicare for All, once again with deceptive disinformation campaigns. We can expect a battle royal over health care all the way through the 2020 election cycle.

There are four key issues involved in the future of U. S. health care:

1. Who is the health care system for—profiteering corporate stakeholders, their shareholders and Wall Street investors—or patients, families, and taxpayers?

2. Is health care just another commodity for sale in our largely for-profit market-based system—or essential services based on medical necessity?

3. Is health care a human right or a privilege based on ability to pay?

4. What ethic should prevail in health care—a business "ethic" maximizing revenue to providers or a service ethic based on needs of patients and their families?

As in other parts of our economy, the GOP-led push toward increasing privatization, based on the discredited meme that "private is better and more efficient," continues to limit access and quality of health care as corporate providers profit on the backs of the sick and the poor. Privatized Medicare and Medicaid serve as examples for this amoral approach to health care.

This book has four goals:

1. To identify and define issues concerning health care reform across the political spectrum in the upcoming 2020 election cycle;
2. To expose disinformation and demagoguery for what it is;
3. To focus on the real stakes for the American people regardless of political ideology; and
4. To help educate policy makers, legislators, and the electorate concerning the real issues and likely outcomes of alternative approaches to health care reform.

As a continuing outlier without universal coverage of health care among virtually all advanced countries, can the U. S. do better? Can we reform our system for the common good, not commercial gain? We all need accessible and affordable essential medical care some times during our lives, often at unpredictable moments. Will anyone be there for us then?

It is my hope that this book will help voters and legislators to better understand the differences among policy alternatives and to support what will best meet the needs of ordinary Americans.

—John Geyman, M.D.
Friday Harbor, WA
May, 2019

PART I

BARRIERS UNDER TRUMPCARE

Something inside the human spirit cries out against the injustice of inequality when you know people who have to choose between food and medicine in a country where CEOs make more in an hour than their lowest-paid employees make in a month.

—The Reverend Dr. Barber II, WJ, president of the North Carolina chapter of the NAACP, pastor at Greenleaf Christian Church in Greensboro, North Carolina, and founder of Repairers of the Breech.

CHAPTER 1

GROWING NUMBERS OF UNINSURED

We have long known that lack of health insurance condemns much of the U. S. population to poor access to essential health care, leading to poor outcomes if and when they ever do receive care. Although the Affordable Care Act (ACA), enacted in 2010, temporarily and partially relieved some of this problem, especially through expansion of Medicaid in many states, it has completely failed to address this ongoing chronic problem in our unfair and cruel health care non-system.

In this chapter we will (1) update the current and projected numbers of being uninsured in America, and (2) describe the impacts experienced by some of the uninsured in gaining access to care.

Current and Projected Numbers of the Uninsured

The best estimates for the number of uninsured in this country are produced by the National Center for Health Statistics of the U.S. Department of Health and Human Services. Here is what we know from its 2018 projections.

- In the first three months of 2018, 28.3 million (8.8 percent) of Americans were uninsured, even eight years after the ACA was initiated. [1]

- This number includes almost 6 million uninsured mothers, one in five are likely to have the greatest physical and mental health care needs. [2]
- One in eight adults between ages 18 to 64 were uninsured.
- Among children from birth to age 17, 5 percent were uninsured. [3]
- One-third of those with family incomes below 200 percent of the federal poverty level (FPL) were uninsured in 2015. [4]
- The 19 states that refused to expand Medicaid under the ACA left 4.8 million people uninsured because of the "Medicaid coverage gap", those with incomes too low to qualify for the ACA's exchanges but above Medicaid eligibility levels. [5]
- An additional 18 million Americans have a gap in insurance coverage at some time during the year, according to the U. S. Census Bureau. [6]

These numbers are all getting worse under the continued efforts by the GOP and Trump administration to sabotage the ACA and cut back on safety net programs.

There are many ways in our current chaotic system whereby people who have health insurance lose that coverage and join the increasing ranks of the uninsured. These are just some of them:

- Loss of a job that provided health insurance.
- Employers stopping previous coverage, very common among small employers.
- Lose employer-sponsored coverage when unable to work because of disability.

- Inability to afford co-payments, deductibles, and co-insurance.
- Becoming "insured" with policies now approved by the Trump administration that exclude essential categories of care that previously were required by the ACA (e.g. short-term plans).
- Losing coverage when dis-enrolled by insurer or insurer exiting the market.
- Previous coverage on parents' insurance under the ACA until aging off at age 26.

Some Barriers to Care Among the Uninsured
Poverty

This patient's experience shows how the above abstract numbers impact real people despite what remains of an increasingly tattered safety net.

> *Sarai was born with Wilson's disease, an inherited disorder that leads to liver failure. She could have been cured by having a liver transplant, but was denied at two prominent liver transplant hospitals in Chicago for lack of insurance coverage. She died at age 25, when her physician signed her death certificate as liver failure. The real cause of her death, however, was inequality.* [7]

Rising inequality within our population has become a massive gulf between the haves and have-nots. Today, in this supposed land of plenty with an annual federal budget of almost $3.5 trillion, 43 million Americans out of our population of 326 million are living in poverty. [8] Unless they can qualify for Medicaid, most will be uninsured, with many millions unable to afford an emergency payment of $400. The 2017 tax bill hailed by the GOP as savings for everyday Americans did nothing of the sort—almost two-thirds of the cuts have gone to the top 20 percent of earners. [9]

A 2012 report by the Centers for Disease Control and Prevention (CDC) estimated that 45,000 Americans are dying each year due to the lack of health insurance. [10] We can expect these numbers to increase as the GOP and Trump administration increase the barriers to affordable health insurance.

Uninsured with income too high for ACA subsidies or Medicaid.

This young man had a tragic outcome being left out of health insurance coverage for his Type 1 diabetes:

Alec R. Smith, 26, aged off from his mother's health insurance plan on his birthday. He had been on insulin for years for Type 1 diabetes. He and his mother explored options over the three months before his birthday. His annual income as a restaurant manager was about $35,000, too high to qualify for Medicaid and also too high to be eligible for subsidies under Minnesota's ACA insurance marketplace. The plan they found [was unaffordable with] a monthly premium of $450 and an annual deductible of $7,600. He hoped to afford his $1,300 monthly bill for diabetes supplies (mostly for insulin) by getting a part-time job. But he died of diabetic ketoacidosis a month later, just three days before payday, having apparently rationed his insulin, with an empty insulin syringe at his side.

The back story is horrific, but telling, as an example of what happens every day to many others. Alec's first vial of insulin cost $24.56 in 2011 after insurance, increasing to $80 in 2018. When he aged off his mother's insurance that year, he could not afford his diabetes supplies. His salary was too high to qualify for Medicaid or Minnesota's health insurance marketplace under the ACA. [11]

Insulin was discovered in the early 1920s by researchers at the University of Toronto, for which Frederick Banting and J. J. R. Macleod received the Nobel Prize in 1923. The patent for this life-saving discovery was sold to the University of Toronto for just $1 so that it could be available for everyone needing it. Where is that humanity today?!

A single vial of insulin now costs more than $250, and most patients use two to four vials each month. [12] The Boston area in Massachusetts has a booming economy in drug companies, including Sanofi, which has marked up prices for its insulin products by as much as 4,500 percent over the estimated cost of producing a single vial of insulin. With insulin no longer affordable, many other patients are dying. Grieving mothers recently led a march against Sanofi, carrying the ashes of their dead children and demanding that the company cut its prices. [13]

Non-acceptance by physicians of patients

Medicaid, of course, is a major part of our existing safety net. Many states impose very restrictive criteria for enrollment, but even if one receives a Medicaid card, the next problem is to find a physician who will accept that coverage. Only about two-thirds of U. S. physicians will accept Medicaid patients, mostly because of very low reimbursement that is typically below the cost of their providing care. Without Medicaid, gaining access to care is even more difficult.

Inadequate care in migrant detention centers

Conditions for medical care under the Trump Administration's immigrant policies at the southern border are abysmal, as these two experiences show:

> *Seeking asylum with her mother, Mariee Juarez as a toddler was detained with her mother at Dilley, Texas, the largest of three family detention centers with 2,400 beds. Although she was in good health on entry, Marilee soon developed high fevers and a worsening respiratory infection. Her care was inadequate. She was never seen by a physician, and was summarily transferred by air with her mother to New Jersey, where she was seen in an emergency room and sent on to hospitals within the area, where she died several weeks later of respiratory failure.* [14]

> *A 7-year-old girl from Guatemala crossed the southern border with her father from Mexico on December 6, 2018. Under custody of the Border Patrol, she had a body temperature of 105.7 degrees eight hours later when she started having seizures. She reportedly had had neither food nor water for several days, and there was no record of her being examined or receiving any care before the onset of her seizures. She was flown by helicopter to Providence Children's Hospital in El Paso, where she was "revived" after a cardiac arrest, but she died less than 24 hours later of septic shock. It took a week for the news of this tragedy to become public.* [15]

These are just two examples of pervasive poor care in family detention centers along the southern border under the Trump administration's Immigration and Customs Enforcement program (ICE). Two physicians, Drs. Scott Allen and Pamela McPherson, under contract to the Department of Homeland Security, have recently issued a scathing report of conditions in these family detention centers, describing freezing conditions, filthy toilets, inadequate water and food, inadequate and untrained staff, and poor medical care. One child lost one-third of his body weight, while an infant with cerebral bleeding went undiagnosed for five days. [16]

Conclusion

We will describe other circumstances in Chapter 4 whereby many other uninsured Americans find themselves in desperate straits without coverage. We need to ask ourselves—is this the America we want to live in? Can't we do better? These unanswered questions will come back to haunt us in all of the following chapters.

References

1. Cohen, RA, Martinez, ME, Zammitti, EP. Health insurance coverage: Early release of estimates from the National Health Interview Survey, January-March 2018. U. S. Department of Health and Human Services. *National Center for Health Statistics*, August 2018.

2. Karpman, M, Gates, K, Kenney, GM et al. How are moms faring under the Affordable Care Act? Evidence through 2014, *Urban Institute*, May 5, 2016.

3.   Scott, D. Under Trump, the number of uninsured kids is suddenly rising. *Vox*, November 29, 2018.

4.   Keenan, PS, Jacobs, PD, Miller, GE. Despite coverage gains, one-third of people in small-firm low-income families were uninsured in 2014-2015. *Health Affairs*, October 2018.

5.   Saloner, B, Hochhalter, W, Sabik, L. Medicaid and CHIP premiums and access to care: A systematic review. *Pediatrics* 137 (3): March 2016.

6.   U. S. Census Bureau, September 2017.

7.   Ansell, D. I watched my patients die of poverty for 40 years. It's time for single-payer. *The Washington Post*, September 13, 2017.

8.   Powers, N. Fear of a black planet: Under the Republican push for welfare cuts, racism boils. *Truthout*, January 21, 2018.

9.   Boushey, H. The tax bill should've been called the Inequality Exacerbation Act of 2017. *The Hill*, December 22, 2017.

10. CDC reports 45,000 die each year for lack of health insurance. *Daily Kos*, October 15, 2012.

11. Sable-Smith, B. Insulin's high cost leads to lethal rationing. *NPR*, September 1, 2018.

12. Altman, D. It's not just the uninsured—it's also the cost of health care. *Axios*, August 20, 2018.

13. Saini, V. As drug prices rise, is Boston's prosperity based on a moral crime? *WBUR*, January 31, 2019.

14. Rose, J. A toddler's death adds to concerns about migrant detention. *NPR*, August 28, 2018.

15. Miroff, N, Moore, R. 7-year-old migrant girl taken into Border Patrol custody dies of dehydration, exhaustion. *The Washington Post*, December 13, 2018.

16. Jordan, M. Whistle-blowers say detaining migrant families 'poses high risk of harm'. *New York Times*, July 18, 2018.

CHAPTER 2

EPIDEMIC OF *UNDER*INSURED

Nine years after passage of the Affordable Care Act (ACA), we still have an epidemic of underinsured Americans. Despite paying more every year for premiums, deductibles, copayments, co-insurance, and out-of-pocket costs, tens of millions of people find themselves without coverage when they need it.

Underinsurance has been defined by the Commonwealth Fund as households spending more than 10 percent of their annual income on health care, not including premiums. The costs of insurance and health care combined have already grown to crisis proportions, with a typical family of four in 2018 paying more than $28,000 a year (including forgone wage increases when insured by their employers). [1] That amount represents nearly 50 percent of the median income for the average family of four of almost $60,000 in 2017.

The ACA did reduce the numbers of uninsured, but more people are underinsured today than in 2010 when it was enacted—87 million, or 45 percent of U. S. adults between the ages of 19 to 64. [2] The gravity of this problem can be better appreciated by knowing that all the trends under TrumpCare *exacerbate* this already serious and unsustainable problem. The GOP and Trump administration have sabotaged the ACA in many ways, including repeal of the individual mandate, weakening of patient protections, relaxing requirements for insurers to cover essential benefits, stopping cost sharing reduction (CSR) payments, and cutbacks to safety net programs such as Medicaid and SNAP (food stamps).

This chapter describes and illustrates with typical patient experiences the many kinds of ways that patients suffer under an increasing burden of being *underinsured*, whether through employer-sponsored health insurance, Medicare, Medicaid, ACA marketplace plans, or other kinds of health insurance.

Underinsurance by Type of Insurance
Employer-sponsored health insurance

A recent national survey by the Commonwealth Fund found that employer-sponsored insurance (ESI) remains the largest single component of health insurance in the U. S., covering about 152 million people, 56 percent of adults under age 65, either through their own or a family member's coverage. But this insurance is increasingly expensive for employers and employees, has more gaps in coverage, and often cannot be relied upon when major illness or accidents occur. [3]

The Kaiser Family Foundation reports that insuring one family in an employer-based plan now costs an average of $19,616 in total annual premiums, of which the worker pays $5,547. These costs have been rising at nearly double recent rates of inflation and increases in workers' pay. Premiums for family plans sponsored by smaller employers have gone up by 55 percent in the last ten years, an unsustainable burden for workers and small employers. [4]

In response to these soaring costs, employers shift more costs to their employees, including ever-increasing deductibles and co-payments when visiting a physician's office or hospital. Some employers are cutting deals directly with private insurers that keep premiums affordable but transfer most costs of health care to their employees if they get sick, and also reduce benefits of their plans. As one example, Meyers Distributing, an auto parts and shipping company based in Indiana, requires its 900 workers to pay $5,000 in annual deductibles ($10,000 for families). Mike Braun, Meyer's CEO, who took a salary from Meyer of $180,000 last year and is worth between $35 and 96 million, defends his plan by saying: "All we've done in my business, and it's not mysterious, is basically harness nature. If you have skin in the game and you feel the cost of something, you shop around". [5]

Privatized Medicare Advantage and Medigap

The private health insurance industry in the U. S. has been increasingly involved and dependent on public programs such as Medicare and Medicaid in recent years. In terms of total industry "net premiums written" (NPW), Medicaid's share grew to 27 percent while Medicare's share increased to 25.5 percent of total overall industry premiums. [6]

CMS unabashedly promotes Medicare Advantage over traditional Medicare in many ways, including shortening the annual open enrollment period, cutting funding for "navigators" who help new enrollees understand and cope with their choices in a timely way, false promises that Medicare Advantage will get extra benefits for less money, and not mentioning the problem of narrow networks which require enrollees to pay much more for out-of-network care.

Traditional public Medicare, of course, provides full choice of physician and hospital anywhere in the country, and with access to a comprehensive set of benefits without networks. Since it covers 80 percent of the costs of physician and hospital care, many patients purchase supplemental Medigap coverage through private insurers.

When they get sick, patients with Medicare Advantage may soon find essential services denied, as happened to this family:

> *John McAuliffe, 77, and his wife, Ann, 78, in Charlotte, NC, were satisfied with their Medicare Advantage plan until she had a severe stroke in 2017. Their insurer refused to pay for further care after several months. While the couple challenged the denial and finally prevailed in a hearing before an administrative law judge, they went back to traditional Medicare and fortunately also obtained a supplemental Medigap policy which together covered all their medical expenses.* [7]

The McAuliffs were fortunate in getting a Medigap plan. Many other sick disenrollees from Medicare Advantage are unable to obtain Medigap coverage for what Medicare does not cover. In fact, seniors on Medicare can be denied a Medigap policy in all but four states because of a pre-existing condition. [8]

Insurers have a symbiotic relationship with the federal government in a number of ways, mostly below the radar for the public to understand. Directories of participating physicians and hospitals in a Medicare Advantage plan are often inaccurate, even including physicians who have died or moved. Despite threats by CMS that it will crack down on these abuses, it never does. [9]

The original agreement in the early 1980s called for private Medicare HMO plans, supposedly more efficient, to receive 95 percent of payments received by original Medicare for fee-for-service care received by beneficiaries in their county of residence. That policy soon markedly changed as a gaming system was launched whereby big overpayments to private plans became the norm—overpayments of about $283 billion between 1985 and 2008 and another $173 billion between 2008 and 2016. [10, 11] The question must be asked—why is this allowed to continue?

The economics of privatized Medicare tell us why insurers welcome gaining market share. Payments to Medicare Advantage plans are based on their risk as reported to the government. This leads them to overstate these risks to get higher payments by up-coding and doing chart reviews to find extra diagnoses. As one example, an insurer of a patient being treated for diabetes without complications may receive an annual payment of $6,765 but if another code is tacked on for vascular disease, that payment increases to $9,796. They game the system in various ways, including by seeking out healthier patients and dis-enrolling them when they get sick, and overstating the severity of their illnesses. Insurers pay for-profit vendors to do chart reviews in order to increase patients' risk scores. One vendor, SCIO Health Analytics, says that its insurer clients gain an average increase in their enrollees' risk scores of 18 percent in the first year and 56 percent in the second year. [12]

While the continued growth of private health insurance at taxpayer expense makes insurers and investors happy, patients and their families so "insured" lose out in many ways, as these examples show:

- Despite advertising for free choice of physician and hospital, most patients soon find themselves with restricted (and changing) networks of available physicians and hospitals in a given plan.
- Sicker people on Medicare Advantage commonly dis-enroll, usually citing restricted access to preferred physicians and hospitals or other medical care. [13]

- A 2017 study in New York State found greater racial health disparities among patients hospitalized with Medicare Advantage compared to traditional Medicare, with black patients receiving worse post-hospital care resulting in higher readmission rates. [14]

Medicaid

The overall thrust of the Trump administration's policies on Medicaid is to reduce and weaken the ACA's Medicaid expansion, and cut back eligibility and enrollment, especially through state waivers. These waivers increase the numbers of people without health insurance by allowing states to impose premiums and other cost sharing, as well as new work requirements; lifetime limits on coverage are also being considered. [15] Mary Mayew has been appointed to head the national Medicaid program and the Children's Health Insurance Program (CHIP). In her former position under outgoing Maine Governor Paul LePage, she boasted of cutting Medicaid enrollment by 24 percent as well as reducing enrollment in the Temporary Assistance for Needy Families program by 70 percent. [6]

Work requirements for Medicaid (20 hours a week) are especially controversial, since studies by the Kaiser Family Foundation tell us that 8 in 10 Medicaid-enrolled nonelderly adults already live in working families and that 60 percent are working themselves. Those who are not working report such obstacles to getting a job as illness, disability, caregiving responsibilities, or being enrolled in school. Meanwhile, of course, implementation of work requirements requires a big increase in bureaucracy to track changing circumstances of enrollees. [17]

As with Medicare Advantage, privatized Medicaid as adopted by a growing number of states also has major downsides:

- Compared to their not-for-profit counterparts, private Medicaid plans have longer waits for care, inadequate physician networks, and denials of many treatments even as insurers take away higher profits. [18]
- Privatized Medicaid programs have worse outcomes than their public counterparts. [19]
- Overpaymants to private Medicaid plans are endemic in more than 30 states, often involving unnecessary or duplicative payments to providers. [20]
- Centene Corp., the largest private Medicaid insurer in the country, took in $1.1 billion in profits between 2014 and 2016 in California, even as its plans were among the worst performing in the state. [21]

ACA marketplace plans

Although the GOP has failed to repeal the ACA on multiple occasions, it has sabotaged it at every turn. The Trump administration has instituted administrative rules and guidance letters intended to undermine the insurance markets, and relaxed many patient protections of the ACA. It has further segmented insurance markets, given private insurers new opportunities to profit from a deregulated marketplace, and pass along higher costs to patients and their families. Among these changes are ACA-exempt short term limited benefit plans with minimal patient protections, association health plans that cross state lines, and insurers now being able to charge seniors premiums that are five times as much as younger people compared to the ACA's 3:1 ratio. [22]

As a result of these waivers, enrollment in ACA's plans has dropped off as their premiums increase in a more divided market where healthier people are separated from the sick within a more fragmented risk pool. ACA enrollees face higher premiums and cost sharing, with many selecting bronze plans that cover only 60 percent of health care costs.

Short-Term Plans

Now that states can circumvent the ACA's patient protections, they can use federal funds to roll out short-term plans with such skimpy benefits as to be labeled "junk insurance." With "coverage" up to a day short of one year, they can be renewed for two more years. They typically exclude coverage of the ACA's ten essential benefits while also denying coverage on the basis of pre-existing conditions. Seema Verma, head of CMS, defends these plans by saying that Trump's goal is to "make health insurance more affordable by expanding choices, increasing competition, reducing federal regulations, and giving states more power to revamp their health insurance market." [23]

A study by the Kaiser Family Foundation of two dozen short-term plans sold in 45 states and the District of Columbia has found that 43 percent had no coverage for mental health services, 62 percent didn't cover substance abuse treatment, 71 percent had no coverage for outpatient prescription drugs, and none covered maternity care. [24]

Short-term plans will yield a bonanza of profits for insurers, who offer them with low premiums and large deductibles. UnitedHealthCare offers plans ranging from one for less than $80 a month with a $12,500 annual deductible to one with a $1,000 deductible for $250 a month. The National Association of Insurance Commissioners has found that insurers paid out an average of just 55 percent of their premiums on actual health care in 2017. [25]

Supplemental indemnity plans

These are very limited plans that target lower-income people with low premiums but provide very poor coverage. Anthem Inc., United Health Group Inc., and Chubb Ltd. offer these plans that make payments toward such services as hospital stays, laboratory tests, and chemotherapy. These insurers admit that these plans are supplemental only and no substitute for comprehensive health insurance. Here is one example of such "coverage":

> *Isaiah Alicea, 29, a refrigeration technician in San Antonio, Texas, purchased a product called Core Health Insurance for just $200 a month. He considered himself healthy, and was aware of just how limited his coverage would be if he got sick—up to $70 each for up to 10 doctor visits, up to $500 a day for a hospital stay up to 31 days, but nothing for hospital care related to pre-existing conditions for the first 12 months that the plan was in effect.* [26]

Conclusion

Continuing false promises for privatized plans under Trump-Care appear to be part of a long-standing conservative agenda to reduce Medicare and Medicaid to small, poorly funded programs while handing over lucrative markets to private insurers with little accountability and ongoing abuses of the public interest. In the next chapter, we will examine how unstable and volatile health insurance has become in this country under the Trump administration.

References:

1. Girod, C, Hart, S, Waltz, S. 2018 *Milliman Medical Index.*
2. Collins, SR, Bhupal, HK, Doty, MM. Health insurance coverage eight years after the ACA. *The Commonwealth Fund*, February 7, 2019.
3. Collins, SR, Radley, DC. The cost of employer insurance is a growing burden for middle-income families. *The Commonwealth Fund*, December 7, 2018.
4. Hancock, J. High-deductible health plans fall from grace in employer-based coverage. *Kaiser Health News*, October 3, 2018.
5. Ollstein, AM. 'It was not real insurance.' *Politico*, October 5, 2018.
6. A. M. Best. *Best's Market Segment Report: U. S. Government-Related Health Insurance Business Continues to Grow Despite Risks*, August 13, 2018.
7. Pear, R. Trump administration peppers inboxes with plugs for private Medicare plans. *New York Times*, December 1, 2018.
8. KFF Newsroom. In all but four states, seniors on Medicare can be denied a Medigap policy due to pre-existing conditions, except during windows of opportunity, July 11, 2018.
9. Cunningham, PW. Trump administration lets Medicare plans off the hook. *The Washington Post*, December 4, 2018.
10. Trivedi, AN, Gribla, RC, Jiang, L et al. Duplicate federal payments to dual enrollees in Medicare Advantage plans and the Veterans Affairs Health Care System. *JAMA* 308 (1) 67-72, 2012.
11. Geruso, M, Layton, T. Upcoding inflates Medicare costs in excess of $2 billion annually. *UT News*, University of Texas at Austin, June 18, 2015.
12. Livingston, S. Insurers profit from Medicare Advantage's incentive to add coding that boosts reimbursement. *Modern Healthcare*, September 4, 2018.
13. Schulte, F. As seniors get sicker, they're more likely to drop Medicare Advantage plans. *Kaiser Health News*, July 6, 2017.
14. Li, Y, Cen, X, Thirukamaran, CP et al. Medicare Advantage associated with more racial disparity than traditional Medicare for hospital readmissions. *Health Affairs*, July 2017.

15. Bernstein, J, Katch, H. Trump administration's under-the-radar attack on Medicaid is gaining speed. *The Washington Post*, March 6, 2018.

16. Diamond, D, Ehley, B. Controversial former aide to Maine's LePage to run Medicaid. *Politico*, October 15, 2018.

17. Rampell, C. Trump is hoping you won't notice his backdoor repeal of Obamacare. *The Washington Post*, January 15, 2018.

18. Himmelstein, DU, Woolhandler, S. The post-launch problem: The Affordable Care Act's persistently high administrative costs. *Health Affairs Blog*, May 27, 2017.

19. McCue, MJ, Bailit, MH. Assessing the financial health of Medicaid managed care plans and the quality of care they provide. New York. *The Commonwealth Fund*, June 15, 2011.

20. Herman, B. Medicaid's unmanaged managed care. *Modern Healthcare*, April 30, 2016.

21. Terhune, C, Gorman, A. Enriched by the poor: California health insurers make billions through Medicaid. *Kaiser Health News*, November 6, 2017.

22. Gluck, AR, Turret, E. The ticking time bomb under Obamacare. *New York Times*, December 6, 2018.

23. Pear, R. Trump officials make it easier for states to skirt Health Law's protections. *New York Times*, October 22, 2018.

24. Cunningham, PW, Firozi, P. The health care world slams Trump's proposal for short-term insurance plans. *The Washington Post*, April 24, 2018.

25. Kodjak, A. Buyer beware: New cheaper insurance policies may have big coverage gaps. *NPR*, October 1, 2018.

26. Matthews, AW. Insurers sell cheaper health plans. *Wall Street Journal*, April 19, 2018: B3

CHAPTER 3

VOLATILITY AND INSTABILITY OF HEALTH INSURANCE

Amidst the ongoing turmoil of a changing marketplace for both public and private health insurance, we can no longer count on our insurance being there when we need it.

This chapter has two goals: (1) to describe and illustrate what Americans are now facing regardless of the kind of health insurance they have; and (2) to briefly consider some of the impacts of losing this coverage.

Across the Board Instability and Volatility
ACA marketplace plans

Inadequate and changing networks are an ongoing problem in this new health care landscape under the Trump administration, which expects 39 states to determine whether health plans sold on the federal insurance exchanges have an adequate number of doctors. There are no real standards for adequacy, and states tend to take a hands-off approach as insurers change their networks on short notice, invariably with the goal to increase their revenues, never with the goal to serve their enrollees by assuring access to quality medical care. For example, nowhere in the equation are such standards as limiting the time and distance that patients should have to travel to access needed care or the need to maintain accurate directories of physicians and hospitals for plans being marketed.

These patient vignettes illustrate what is going on across the country, revealing the lack of standards and patient protections under TrumpCare.

Cynthia Harvey, a resident in Spokane, Washington, purchased an insurance plan from Coordinated Care, which promised a robust roster of physicians and coverage for an array of services, including emergency room coverage if needed. A federal lawsuit, however, soon revealed that Coordinated Care, owned by its parent company, Centene Corporation, had no emergency room physicians in its network at the time of her enrollment. When she had to see an out-of-network emergency room physician, she was confronted by a $1,544 bill.

Steven Milman, a Texas periodontist in Austin, Texas, enrolled in Superior Health, a health plan also owned by Centene Corporation, after reading on its website that Superior included the 140 physicians of the Austin Diagnostic Clinic in its provider network. After the above lawsuit against Centene, he learned that the Austin Diagnostic Clinic had informed Superior some months earlier that it would no longer accept Superior patients. After a long delay and many entreaties from Dr. Milman, Superior finally assigned him a primary care physician—an obstetrician-gynecologist! [1]

In many instances, preferred hospitals are excluded from insurers' networks, even when enrollees have had previous care in these hospitals. This problem is even worse for highly specialized academic medical centers, which provide care for the sickest and most costly patients, as this example shows:

Christopher Briggs, a self-employed communications consultant for nonprofit groups, his wife and four-year old child, Colette, live in Loudoun County, Virginia. The family has had health insurance through Anthem for years. Colette had been in and out of chemotherapy treatments at Inova Fairfax Hospital since age two for leukemia until the insurer stopped selling policies in Virginia. Pressure from the state resumed coverage in some counties and cities, but the family's zip code was not among them. The only insurer available to them was Cigna, which does not cover Fairfax Hospital, the only local hospital with a dedicated pediatric cancer unit where she has received all of her care for leukemia. Desperate for continued coverage of Colette's specialized care, Christopher was forced to consider moving his 11-person family to another zip code, or even to give up his solo business and go back to working for someone else. Initial pleas to Cigna for an exception were not responsive. [2]

Employer-sponsored health insurance

Although more than one-half of American adults under age 65 have employer-sponsored health insurance, as individuals or families, this coverage can be very unreliable, as this patient experienced.

Stephanie Burdick, 30, a resident of West Jordan, Utah, suffered a traumatic brain injury at age 27 while surfing in California when her head struck another surfer's board. She was hospitalized for almost a month and had to relearn how to talk, walk, and most other activities. She lost her health insurance when her former employer realized that she wouldn't be able to return to work soon. Her bare-bones plan excluded essential treatments, including those for a walking and balance therapist, neuro-ophthalmologist, speech therapist, and treatment for migraine headaches. She applied for Medicaid, but couldn't receive that care until it was approved 19 months later. [3]

Medicare Advantage

As we saw in the last chapter, insurers have many ways to game industry friendly policies of the Trump administration. Private Medicare Advantage has more than doubled since 2010 to more than 20 million enrollees, a quarter of Medicare beneficiaries, and growing. There are now about 3,700 private plans which are expected to enroll almost 23 million people in 2019. As a result of federal overpayments through gamed risk-adjustments and bonuses that have nothing to do with quality monitoring, insurers can offer extra benefits, such as vision and dental coverage, and still make lots of money. [4]

As we would expect, however, the tradeoffs for seniors are detrimental in many ways, especially through narrow networks that restrict choice and denial of services. A recent report by the Inspector General of DHHS found "widespread and persistent problems related to denials of care and payment through Medicare Advantage." The report also found "onerous and often unnecessary pre-authorization requirements," barriers to timely access to care, and annual limits on out-of-pocket costs (that traditional Medicare does not have). Denial of services keeps down insurers' costs and increases their profits. Medicare has imposed more than $10 million in fines against these plans in the last two years without changing this pattern of violations. Incredibly, the government does not even include audit violations in its star quality rating system! [5]

Medicaid

Medicaid coverage has become more and more tenuous under the Trump administration's policies discussed in the last chapter. Here is one typical example of unpredictable changes of contracts between private Medicaid plans and provider institutions that leave patients in the lurch.

> *Lee Henderson has been a patient at U. C. Davis Medical Center since childhood. Because of severe elevations of his blood pressure, he needed to have surgery to remove his adrenal gland. He was covered by Health Net at that time, the only Medi-Cal managed care plan in Sacramento County whose members could go to U. C. Davis for primary care. Shortly before planned surgery, however, the insurer and the university terminated their contract, forcing him and about 3,700 other Health Net Medi-Cal members to leave U. C. Davis and find new primary care physicians. He did have surgery there in 2015, and regained access to U. C. Davis in 2017 when UnitedHealthcare entered the Sacramento Medi-Cal market. But history repeated itself in 2018, when UnitedHealthcare notified its members, with just three months' notice, that its services in Sacramento would soon be discontinued.* [6]

Arkansas was the first state to require Medicaid enrollees to prove to the state that they are working 20 hours a week or 80 hours a month. But that process is so difficult that 80 percent of enrollees make no reports at all. They cannot report directly by phone, by mail, or in person. Their reports must be online, even though Arkansas has the lowest level of household Internet access in the country and the state's website closes down every night from 9 p.m. to 7 a.m. for scheduled maintenance. Moreover, the online portal does not work well with smart phones. As a result, 18,000 Arkansans have lost Medicaid coverage due to these barriers or not understanding or being able to cope with the reporting process. This is how tenuous coverage is for one working Medicaid patient.

Anna Book is homeless and works as a restaurant dishwasher, usually just meeting the state's 80-hour work requirement. She doesn't have a computer, and has designated a pastor to log her work hours for her. If business is light, she might lose a shift at the restaurant. She dropped below the 80-hour minimum once. If that happens two more times, she'll lose her coverage. [7]

These two patient vignettes reveal how tight budgets are for so many millions of patients on Medicaid while limiting their capacity to afford basic necessities of life.

Mark Coleman, 49, a diabetic who had received care at a busy clinic run by Family Health Centers in Kentucky, lost his Medicaid coverage after forgetting to report a change of income the previous year when he switched from a higher-paying job at an Amazon warehouse to a less physically demanding job as a parts driver for Pep Boys, the automotive chain, working 20 hours each week. He has diabetic neuropathy of his hands and feet, and sometimes has trouble walking. Returning to his usual clinic, he was told that Medicaid coverage would soon be reinstated, and his four essential medications were refilled for a month. He admitted that he, his wife and four children often have trouble paying for food, and utilities. He supports work requirements, but faces a personal dilemma—whether or not he should cut back his hours and try to get himself qualified as "medically frail," thereby becoming exempt from the work rules.

Sheila Penny, 54, plagued by chronic depression and anxiety since age 16, has worked at various jobs over the years, including as a package handler, a boat reservations manager, and even as a navigator helping patients to sign up for Medicaid. Her mother has paid her rent for the last two years as she has tried to get herself to a better place mentally. She expects to be able to pay the new $4 per month premiums for Medicaid in Kentucky, but does admit that she wonders if she can also pay for dog food. [8]

Emergency room care

With the intent to rein in emergency room costs, some insurers are calling some such visits avoidable and refusing coverage for them. Anthem denied thousands of these claims in 2017 under its 'avoidable' E.R. program, according to an analysis by the American College of Emergency Physicians. Here is one such example of many:

- *Jim Burton, 37, felt a jolt in his back that dropped him to his knees instantly when lifting a box in his garage. He thought he had slipped a disc. A friend, also an emergency medical technician, urged him to go to the hospital. After assessment in an E. R., he was sent home with a diagnosis of "back sprain." His insurer, Anthem, refused to pay for his medical bills totaling $1,722, with the statement that "his E. R. care was not necessary to avoid a serious risk to health." Jim appealed that decision, and Anthem finally paid.* [9]

Anthem, with almost 40 million enrollees across the country, rolled out this policy in six states, and was soon sued by the American College of Emergency Physicians and the Medical Association of Georgia. This practice is another example of insurer greed. Senators Claire McCaskill of Missouri and Ben Cardin of Maryland sent a letter in protest to DHHS stating that "by denying patient claims based on the patient's final diagnosis and ignoring the patient's symptoms present at the time of the emergency, we believe that Anthem likely violated federal law." [10]

Women's health care

An escalating war on women has been waged by conservative Republicans and the Trump administration that knows no bounds and rips apart a long history of protections for women over the last 50 years. The Title X Family Planning Program was enacted under President Richard Nixon in 1970, while the U. S. Supreme Court decriminalized abortion in its 1973 Roe v. Wade decision. Today's pro-life forces are dedicated to overturning that decision. GOP efforts to defund Planned Parenthood continue, together with closure of many such clinics in many states. Trump signed an executive order in 2017 that allows employers with a moral or religious objection to stop insurance coverage for contraceptive services, as has been required by the ACA, that can affect up to 62 million people.

Today, the Trump administration has relaxed the ACA's requirement to cover ten essential services. Short-term and other new plans typically exclude coverage of maternity care and preventive services. Trump's recently proposed Title X rule would impose a gag rule on discussing abortion by Planned Parenthood caregivers, thereby disrupting access to contraception, cancer screenings, and treatment of sexually transmitted diseases for some 4 million patients. In response, the ACLU has joined with a powerful coalition of partner organizations and 21 states attorney generals in filing suit over this policy. [11]

These policies make no sense, and are detrimental to women, their families, and our society for a number of reasons:

- According to the Guttmacher Institute, 70 percent of women in their childbearing years (15 to 44) are at risk of unintended pregnancy in being sexually active and not desiring to become pregnant; only 2 percent of Catholic women rely on natural family planning through the rhythm method. Aided by improved birth control and women's access to Planned Parenthood clinics across the country, the U. S. abortion rate dropped to an historic low in 2014. [12]

- Ninety-seven percent of Planned Parenthood services are for preventive services such as contraception options, breast exams, screening for cervical cancer and sexually transmitted infections, with only 3 percent for abortion. [13]

- The hypocrisy of these policies are obvious in this observation by Dr. Hal Lawrence, CEO of the American College of Obstetricians and Gynecologists:

The strange thing about this is that people who want to decrease the number of abortions are taking away access to the very services that help prevent them. [14]

Why are these hurtful policies to American women and their families allowed to continue, especially when we consider that 53 percent of the electorate in our supposed democracy are women and that more than 90 percent of Catholic women use contraception!?

Mental health coverage

Our system for mental health care is completely broken, even for people fortunate enough to have health insurance. Many insurers exclude mental health services from their policies under TrumpCare. Plans that do include mental health coverage typically have inadequate numbers of psychiatrists and other mental health providers in their networks. Many psychiatrists and psychologists in the U. S. will not accept new patients with mental health problems, partly because of low reimbursement that doesn't cover their costs. Just under one-quarter of all psychiatrists in a given area participate in an average insurer's provider network. [15] Despite the supposed health insurance reform under the Romney administration in Massachusetts in 2006 that required state residents to have health insurance, more than one-half of adults who sought mental health or addiction treatment in late 2018 had difficulty getting care, with 39 percent going without treatment. [16]

Here is one example of the parents of a teenager with schizophrenia trying to deal with gaining access to care, despite their being insured.

Joey Hudy started having delusions and paranoia in early 2017. His parents soon found that almost all of the possible treatment centers were out of network or out of state. They had to pay tens of thousands of dollars out-of-pocket to cover the costs of Joey's treatment, with no relief in sight. [17]

The Mental Health Parity and Addiction Equity Act of 2008 required health plans to cover mental health services at least as generously as for medical/surgical services. However, a wide gulf of coverage remains today, and the stigma about mental illness still exists. Almost one in five Americans have had some kind of mental illness or addiction disorder in the past year. Because of lack of access to care, many end up in jail as mental health problems become criminalized. This patient's story exposes the extent of this broken system:

> *Edward Vega, 47, was taking medications for bipolar disorder and schizophrenia until he ran out of them and was arrested in August 2017 on suspicion of drug possession. He was convicted and spent five months in the San Diego County jail. He was hearing voices in his head when admitted to jail and knew that he was going to hurt someone if he didn't get medication. He assaulted a fellow inmate a week later and ended up in isolation, which made him feel worse. Finally, his medications were resumed. He was much improved three months after being released from jail, though he was still hearing some voices.* [18]

Impacts of Losing Health Care Coverage

As we see, health insurance in this country has become increasingly volatile and unstable, especially in this new era under the Trump administration's deregulation of insurers and cutbacks of public programs. Although employer-sponsored health insurance is still the largest source of coverage, it too is more unstable all the time. The Bureau of Labor Statistics estimates that Americans hold an average of twelve different jobs between the ages of 18 and 50, with varying levels of insurance coverage if at all.

A recent study of the impacts of loss of health insurance among people with Type 1 diabetes shows how hazardous interruptions in coverage are. Since they all depend on insulin treatment and close follow-up over the long-term with this chronic disease, they are especially vulnerable to lack or lapses of insurance coverage. This study found that one in four patients had at least one interruption in coverage over an average of 2.6 years. During these times, they needed many more acute care services, more ER visits, and hospitalizations. [19] We can expect worse outcomes for patients with many other diseases who have to deal with interruptions of insurance coverage.

Conclusion

The first three chapters have shown how access to care suffers whether uninsured, underinsured, or insured with volatile and unstable coverage. This takes us to the next chapter, where we will examine how difficult it has become for Americans to afford health insurance that deserves the name "insurance."

References:

1. Ollove, M. Trump administration: Let states decide if health plans have enough doctors. *The Pew Charitable Trust*, February 6, 2018.
2. Itkowitz, AC. Parents of 4-year-old with cancer can't buy ACA plan to cover her hospital care. *The Washington Post*, November 15, 2017.
3. Caldwell, P. Medicaid mutiny: Will red states vote to expand Obamacare? *Mother Jones*, November/December 2018, p. 42.
4. Galewitz, P. Medicare Advantage riding high as new insurers flock to sell to seniors. *Kaiser Health News*, October 15, 2018.

5. Pear, R. Medicare Advantage plans found to improperly deny many claims. *New York Times*, October 13, 2018.

6. Waters, R. Whipsawed: Low-income patients at UC Davis losing coverage again. *California Healthline*, September 26, 2018.

7. Rampell, C. Arkansas's Medicaid experiment has proved disastrous. *The Washington Post*, November 20, 2018.

8. Goodnough, A. Kentucky rushes to remake Medicaid as other states prepare to follow. *New York Times*, February 10, 2018.

9. Abelson, R, Sanger-Katz, M, Creswell, J. As an insurer resists paying for 'avoidable' E. R. visits, patients and doctors push back. *New York Times*, May 19, 2018.

10. Tracer, Z. Anthem sued by doctors in dispute over emergency-room coverage. *Bloomberg News*, July 17, 2018.

11. Dalven, J. We're in the fight of our lives to keep our abortion rights. *American Civil Liberties Union*, March 12, 2019.

12. Dreweke, J. Anti-choice Republicans likely to ignore key reason for abortion rate decline. *Guttmacher Institute*, January 17, 2017.

13. Alonzo-Zaldivar, R, Crary, D. Trump remaking federal policy on women's reproductive health. *Associated Press*, May 30, 2018.

14. Lawrence, H. As quoted in Corbett, J. 'Crisis no one is talking about': GOP threatens health care of 26 million people. *Common Dreams*, February 2, 2018.

15. Andrews, M. Narrow networks get even tighter when shopping for mental health specialists. *Kaiser Health News*, September 22, 2017.

16. Kowalczyk, L. Even with insurance, getting mental health treatment is a struggle in Mass., study says. *Boston Globe*, December 11, 2018.

17. Kennedy, PJ. Insurance system still discriminates against mental illness. Time to fight back. *USA Today*, October 3, 2018.

18. Gorman, A. Use of psychiatric drugs soars in California jails. *Kaiser Health News*, May 8, 2018.

19. Rogers, MAM, Lee, JM, Tipirneni, R et al. Interruptions in private health insurance and outcomes in adults with Type 1 diabetes: A longitudinal study. *Health Affairs*, July 2018.

CHAPTER 4

"I CAN'T AFFORD INSURANCE" STARK CHOICES AND TRADEOFFS DUE TO UNAFFORDABLE HEALTH INSURANCE

There are so many ways that patients and families find themselves in jeopardy of losing insurance that provides them any protection.

The goals of this chapter are: (1) to summarize the relentless rise in costs of health insurance with less and less coverage; and (2) to describe many varied circumstances as patients and families struggle to get some kind of insurance, together with the tradeoffs involved.

Increasing Costs of Health Insurance: An Overview

The costs of health insurance in this country have been rising at rates way above the inflation rate or cost of living for many years. As a result, the costs of insurance and actual health care now consume almost one-half of the average household income for families of four, an unsustainable financial hardship for middle income families.

As the Trump administration sabotaged the ACA, insurers became more uncertain of the markets and their profits, leading to big increases in premiums for 2018—116 percent increase in Arizona and more than 50 percent in other states. Many insurers exited the market, leaving many counties with just one insurer, partly as a result of Trump's discontinuance of cost sharing reduction (CSR) payments in 2017.

The ACA's marketplace set up four levels of coverage, the so-called "metals," with varying actuarial values, costs and coverage: platinum (90 percent coverage), gold (80 percent), silver (70 percent and the benchmark plan), and bronze (60 percent). CSRs were intended to reimburse insurers for their costs in insuring low-income enrollees with incomes up to 250 percent of the federal poverty level. These subsidies were based on the second lowest marketplace plan, the silver benchmark plan. Their discontinuation led to silver plan premiums going up by 7 to 38 percent for 2018, with the average silver plan 75 percent higher than in 2014, according to an analysis by the Kaiser Family Foundation. Unless they can qualify for a government subsidy, the average family of four with 40-year-old parents can expect to pay more than $19,000 in 2019 for the cheapest silver premium in Memphis, Tennessee. Figure 4.1 shows changes in ACA marketplace premiums for 2019 by state. [1]

Premium increases for 2019 are lower than for 2018, dropping by an average of almost 1 percent across all states for the average silver "benchmark" plan that the government uses to set subsidies. That led Trump to falsely claim that his policies were making insurance more affordable. Cynthia Cox, who monitors the ACA marketplaces for the Kaiser Family Foundation, instead wrote: "One big reason insurers are lowering premiums: individual insurers are currently so profitable it would be hard for many companies to justify a rate increase." [2] However, the consulting firm Avalere Health estimated that 2019 premiums would go up in three states—by 69 percent in Iowa, 65 percent in Wyoming, and 64 percent in Utah. [3]

FIGURE 4.1

CHANGES IN KEY ACA MARKETPLACE PREMIUMS FOR 2019

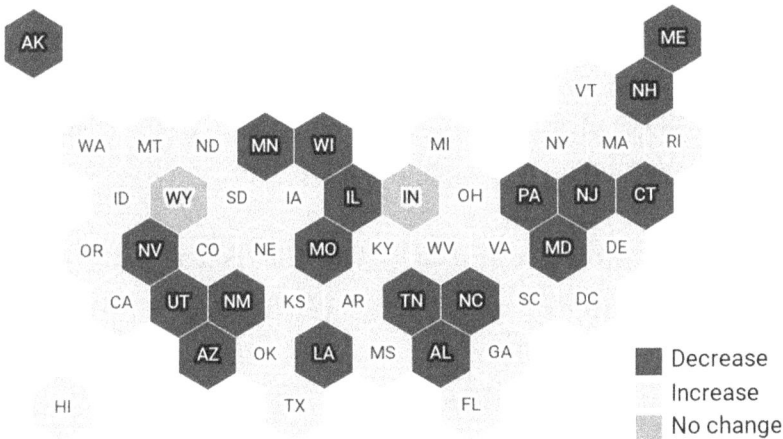

Source: Kaiser Family Foundation Health Tracking Poll, August 23 - 28, 2018

Insurers lure enrollees by trying to make their premiums seem attractive without looking hard at coverage. But patients need to carefully assess coverage, not just premiums, to have any sense of what protection a given plan may or may not provide. The picture is not bright when they do so. The Robert Wood Johnson Foundation has found that less than one-third of plans in the individual market (as opposed to employer-sponsored insurance) offer out-of-network (OON) coverage, that deductibles for 30 percent of plans with OON coverage are more than $20,000, and that there is *no limit* for maximum out-of-pocket (MOOP) costs in one-third of these plans. [4]

Trump's charade of making health insurance more affordable is just another weave of lies. Through waivers to states, new guidelines from the Trump administration will allow federal subsidies to offer skimpier, cheaper plans that don't meet the ACA's requirements, such as patient protections of pre-existing conditions and coverage of ten essential benefits. [5] Short-term plans up to one year, renewable for two years, will be bare bones at most, will not be available to anyone with significant health problems, and will draw healthier people out of the risk pool. The more fragmented the risk pool becomes, the more expensive coverage will be for older, sicker people. Dean Baker, co-director of the Center for Economic and Policy Research, observes:

> *A couple earning $65,000 a year could easily find themselves paying more than half of their after-tax income for insurance premiums. And they could still find themselves liable for thousands of dollars in health care expenses.* [6]

The fact is—private health insurers continue to thrive on the backs of patients, families, and taxpayers as they seek ever higher profits without public accountability. The Kaiser Family Foundation found that insurers in the individual market performed better financially in the first six months of 2018 than they have in all of the years since the ACA was enacted in 2010. [7] In the third quarter of 2018, UnitedHealth, the parent of the country's largest health insurer as well as Optum, its growing health services arm, reported an increase of its net income of 28 percent compared to that of the previous year. [8] Nor can consumers find any help from the 2017 tax bill passed by Trump and the GOP. Almost two-thirds of those tax cuts went to the top 20 percent of Americans, CEO compensation increased by 18 percent and average worker compensation grew by just 0.2 percent. [9]

Varied Circumstances, Options and Tradeoffs to Get and Keep Insurance

People can enroll in bronze ACA plans without having to pay premiums but with big downsides

Many low-income people can get a bronze level plan on the ACA market without any out-of-pocket premiums if they qualify for federal subsidies. In more than 2,500 counties in 2019, the ACA's premium tax credits will fully cover these premiums for a 40-year-old enrollee earning $20,000 a year; in 120 counties, that 40-year-old with an annual income of $40,000 would also pay no premiums. Attractive as that may sound, these plans may turn out to be very expensive, with out-of-pocket and deductibles up to $7,900 a year as well as just 60 percent coverage of health care costs. Figure 4.2 shows counties across the country where these plans are available in 2019. [10]

FIGURE 4.2

COUNTIES WHERE THE LOWEST-COST BRONZE PLAN PREMIUM COSTS ZERO DOLLARS AFTER TAX CREDIT IN 2019

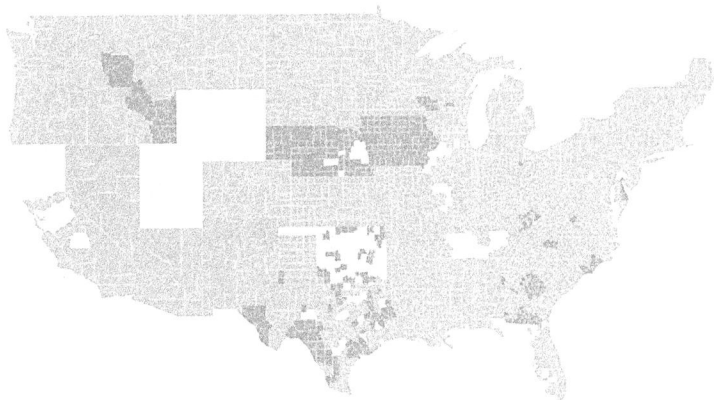

LCB premium fully covered by tax credit (new in 2019)
LCB premium fully covered by tax credit in both 2018 and 2019
LCB premium is higher than amount of tax credit in 2019

Source: Kaiser Family Foundation

This is how a bronze plan works out for one family living just outside Phoenix, Arizona:

> *Theresa Flood, 59, a preschool teacher, lives with her husband John, a pastor, and looked at all of the available plans. Theresa needed ongoing care for spine problems, with a history of four surgeries, and for a cyst and benign brain tumor. The only plan they could afford was a bronze plan that excluded her two specialists. The couple qualified for a $1,263-a-month subsidy that reduced their monthly premiums to $207 a month, but with a $6,550 per person deductible.*[11]

Many individuals drop insurance due to unaffordable costs and loss of in-network coverage

This couple's experience shows how important it is for many people to have in-network coverage for physicians and hospitals of their choice:

> *Dianna Buchanan, 51, survived a bout with cancer 15 years ago, and her husband, Keith, 48, has high blood pressure and takes testosterone shots. Residents of Marion, North Carolina, their annual income from his small IT business and her job as a physical therapy assistant is more than $127,000 a year, plus some income from properties that they own. But they still can't afford health insurance when their annual premium for their policy with Blue Cross and Blue Shield of North Carolina went up to $21,756, with $5,000 per-person deductibles, thereby totaling more than $30,000 a year to retain and use their coverage. At the time they needed to decide about insurance, their hospital of choice had not yet agreed to be in-network, so they were forced to terminate their coverage.*[12]

Many families can't afford insurance because of the 'family glitch'

There was an unfortunate problem built into the ACA, now termed the "family glitch", which is still little known and affects some 6 million people.

Eligibility for federal subsidies was intended for people that didn't have access to affordable health insurance through their employers—determined by having to pay more than 9.86 percent of the family's income—considering only the cost of insuring *one* family member, even if other family members would be so covered. Here is how that obscure rule adversely impacted one typical family trying to deal with this problem.

Justine Bradford-Trent, 54, was uninsured when she slipped on the ice on Christmas eve of 2017. Slamming to the ground, her elbow soon swelled up, and she wondered if it was broken. She and her family were uninsured because of the "family glitch." She debated whether to go to the ER. An urgent care center would have been cheaper, but was closed for the holiday. The Idaho resident decided to wait; after the swelling subsided, she assumed that it was just a bad bruise.

The reasons for their being uninsured were complicated. Her husband works in commercial construction, earning $66,000 a year as the family's primary breadwinner. Justine works part-time as a notary public, earning a few hundred dollars a month, not enough to pay for insurance. To add Justine and their daughter to their plan would cost $718 a month more, a total of $1,060 a month or 25 percent of her husband's take-home pay, not including out-of-pocket costs of any medications or procedures. They decided to just add their daughter to the plan with Justine going uninsured and hoping to stay healthy. [13]

Some families have to choose which family members to drop from small employer coverage

Soaring costs of insurance and health care in this country have forced many small employers to discontinue coverage of their employees and to insure only some family members. This family's experience illustrates the burdens and difficult choices they confronted despite being initially a prosperous middle-class, hard-working family.

David and Maribel Maldonado were the very defini-tion of achieving the American dream. Both immigrated from Mexico, as David's father had done when David was a small child. His father supported his wife and ten chil-dren by working long hours as a mechanic. When David had a family of his own, he was earning about $113,000 a year as a salesman by the time his two children were in their teens. His wife Maribel worked as a hair stylist while caring for their two children. They lived in a nice suburban house outside Dallas, Texas. They had a family insurance plan through David's small welding business with less than a dozen employees.

Then their world came crashing down after Maribel had a double mastectomy for breast cancer in 2012. After two years of Maribel's very expensive treatments and re-covery, David could no longer afford his small employer in-surance policy. Alternate coverage would cost him $1,375 a month, far more than the $260 a month that he had been paying. The family's new insurance plan was costing them almost $23,000 a year, more than they were paying for their mortgage. College expenses were looming as their daughter,

Alexa, was soon to enter college with a long-term goal of becoming a nurse. Of the four, Maribel and Alexa needed the most care, Alexa for asthma, so David decided on the basis of "who got sick the most" to drop himself and their son, Cristian, from the policy, which reduced the monthly premium to $750, still with a $5,000 annual deductible.

There was worse to come. Blue Cross Blue Shield then increased their monthly premium from $750 to $1,060. By then the family was running a monthly deficit of $500 to $600 as Maribel was taking daily tamoxifen and Alexa's asthma hadn't improved. After going to an alternative medicine clinic in Houston, Alexa's asthma improved, to the point that David was able to take her off the family's insurance plan, leaving just Maribel covered. To economize, David gave blood every four or five months to check on his blood pressure, which has been high for several years, and Cristian avoids going to doctors. After all this turmoil and financial hardship, David, who has dual citizenship, considered going to Mexico for care, but this would be an 8 to 9-hour drive. Despite his successful working life, he has to struggle to pay the bills, as the family realizes their vulnerability of an unexpected medical emergency. [14]

Individuals may have incomes too high to qualify for ACA subsidies, but still can't afford health insurance

Under the ACA, people with annual incomes up to 400 percent of the federal poverty level (about $48,500 for an individual and $100,400 for a family of four in 2019), are eligible for premium subsidies. People with higher incomes are on their own, but their costs of health insurance are still high and may not be affordable, as this family found out.

Cameron and Lori Llewellyn, of Dover, Delaware, have had a difficult time affording and keeping health insurance. Cameron is a self-employed construction contractor. In order to start her own business in 2017, a clothing boutique, Lori left her job in 2017 that provided health insurance for their family, including their daughter Bryce. They looked for a plan on the ACA's marketplace, but found a plan with monthly premiums of $2,000 with deductibles of $4,000 or more too expensive and elected to go without coverage. Their incomes were too high to qualify for ACA subsidies. In 2019, they tried again for a plan on the the state exchange. They were fortunate to find a policy with monthly premiums of $1,286 and a $7,900 deductible, together with a subsidy that would cover the entire premium. [15]

Major question: what happens with the legal challenge to the ACA?

In mid-December, 2018, Judge Reed O'Connor in Fort Worth, Texas, ordered a 55-page ruling in a district court that could threaten the survival of the ACA in its entirety if higher courts uphold that it is unconstitutional in requiring an individual mandate. As the latest GOP attempt to unravel the ACA, this could throw the entire health care system into chaos if it is ever held to be unconstitutional, as many observers think unlikely but possible. In response, a group of state Democratic attorneys general has promised to appeal this decision, which would send it to the 5th Circuit Court of Appeals, and possibly, even to the U. S. Supreme Court.

More than 20 million Americans without health insurance gained coverage through the ACA from 2010 to 2017. Important patient protections were provided, such as banning insurers from denying coverage because of pre-existing conditions. More than 30 states expanded Medicaid under the ACA, which also allowed adult children to stay on their parents' health plans until reaching age 26. Despite attacks by the GOP, the ACA enjoys very high levels of public support. Its loss would cause millions of Americans to lose health insurance, adversely impact Medicare and Medicaid, and even set back other important programs, such as the authority of the Center for Medicare & Medicaid Innovation (CMMMI), which was created by the ACA to rein in drug prices. [16]

Here is just one of many examples of how serious the loss of the ACA would be for many millions of Americans.

Kathy Tomasic, 59, is one of 60 percent of Americans with one of her family members with a pre-existing condition. Her son, Alec, has a rare genetic disorder called mastocytosis, which periodically sends his body into shock and lands him in a hospital. Now 15 years old, he is a childhood prodigy, already accepted at the University of California Berkeley with a goal of focusing on fusion research. He gets a monthly shot costing $2,000 in an effort to stabilize his condition. With the ACA, he can stay on his father's insurance until age 26, but if the ACA goes away, he would likely become uninsured at age 19. She needed to move from San Diego, where she had a full-time job with benefits, to Berkeley when Alec moved there. She was able to get a flexible, part-time job there, unfortunately without benefits, but she knew she could get coverage under the ACA with subsidies for its $400 a month premiums. The ACA remains the only available way that she can continue with her family's health and financial security. [17]

Conclusion

Unfortunately, these patient stories are all too common across our cruel and flawed health care non-system. In the next chapter, we will shift our attention to the inability of a growing part of our population to afford actual health care.

References

1. Rau, J. In health insurance wastelands, rosier options crop up for 2019. *Kaiser Health News*, November 23, 2018.

2. Galewitz, P, Appleby, J. Obamacare premiums dip for first time. Some call it a correction. *Kaiser Health News*, October 11, 2018.

3. Milbank, D. Trump just told the truth. He may wish he hadn't. *The Washington Post*, December 20, 2017.

4. Robert Wood Johnson Foundation. To infinity and beyond: Exposure to out-of-network bills is high and rising in the individual and small group markets. October 4, 2018.

5. Hackman, M. States can waive more ACA rules. *Wall Street Journal*, October 23, 2018.

6. Baker, D. Trump succeeds in making insurance for people with health problems unaffordable. *The Progressive Populist*, October 1, 2018, p. 11.

7. Hellmann, J. Study: Insurers returning to pre-Obamacare profitability. *The Hill*, October 5, 2018.

8. Mathews, AW, Chin, K. UnitedHealth boosts earning outlook. *Wall Street Journal*, October 17, 2018: B2.

9. Corn, D. The midterms will determine whether Donald Trump's two-year assault on democratic norms will be repudiated—or validated. *Mother Jones*, November/December, 2018.

10. *Kaiser Family Foundation.* Some can get marketplace plans with no premiums, though with higher deductibles and cost sharing, November 26, 2018.
11. Ibid # 1.
12. Tozzi, J. Why some Americans are risking it and skipping insurance. *Bloomberg*, March 26, 2018.
13. Luthra, S. Fixing Obamacare's 'family glitch' hinges on outcomes of November elections. *Kaiser Health News*, October 23, 2018.
14. Kasumov, A. Soaring health care costs forced this family to choose who can stay insured. *Bloomberg*, November 13, 2018.
15. Findlay, S. Health insurance costs crushing many people who don't get federal subsidies. *Kaiser Health News*, December 14, 2018.
16. Rovner, J. 5 ways nixing the Affordable Care Act could upend the entire health system. *Kaiser Health News*, December 20, 2018.
17. Rampell, C. Republicans' relentless attempts to undermine Obamacare escalate American anxiety. *The Washington Post*, December 18, 2018.

CHAPTER 5

"EVEN WITH HEALTH INSURANCE, I CAN'T AFFORD CARE"

As we saw in the last two chapters, today's market for health insurance has become volatile and unstable as patients and their families pay more and get less coverage. In this chapter, we have two goals to better understand the stakes facing Americans trying to gain access to affordable care: (1) to outline the main drivers of health care costs; and (2) to illustrate with patient stories some of the many ways that people, even with health insurance, still can't deal with the costs of care.

The Main Drivers of Soaring Health Care Costs

Total spending for U. S. health care now exceeds $3 trillion, more than $10,700 per capita. [1] A recent study comparing the U. S. with 10 high-income countries found that we spend almost twice as much on medical care while performing less well on many population health outcomes. Uncontrolled prices were considered to be the main driving factors for spiraling health care costs, especially prices of labor and goods, including pharmaceuticals, medical devices, and administrative costs. [2]

When we look further into our vast medical-industrial complex, we can readily see a number of inter-related trends that make cost containment of health care costs impossible without major financing reform. Here are just some of them.

1. Increasing corporatization and privatization of health care

Corporatization and growth of for-profit health care have been rapidly increasing in recent decades as the ties with Wall Street become ever more intertwined. The so-called "business ethic" puts CEO compensation and shareholders far above the needs of patients. As could be expected, the ACA did not change this situation in any way. CEOs of the largest U. S. health care companies have taken in almost $10 billion since it was passed in 2010.[3] Tom Scully, former administrator of CMS in the George W. Bush administration, saw this coming in these words:

> *Obamacare is not a government takeover of medicine. It is the privatization of health care . . . It is going to make some people very rich.* [4]

In every case, privatization brings higher costs, less efficiency, more bureaucracy, and less service. As their inefficiencies mount, private companies and contractors keep coming back to the government and taxpayers for more support. The extent of privatized ownership is more extensive than most of us may realize—specialty hospitals, 37 percent; nursing homes, 65 percent; home care, 76 percent; dialysis centers, 90 percent; surgi-centers, 96 percent; and free-standing lab/imaging centers, 100 percent. [5]

2. Consolidation and mergers

The growing number of mergers and consolidation, especially among hospital systems, private insurers, pharmaceutical and other industries, result in massive forces for profits over service. As giant corporate systems buy up hospitals and physicians' practices at an increasing rate, they gain market share to near monopoly levels and can set prices to what the traffic will bear. [6] As hospital systems get larger, they invariably increase their prices and patients pay more. [7] In an effort to discourage the use of less expensive rivals, larger hospitals frequently make secret deals with private insurers that add fees and hide prices from consumers. [8]

3. Administrative waste

Administrative costs are estimated to account for 25 to 31 percent of total health expenditures in this country, twice that in Canada and much higher than in other OECD countries. Almost two-thirds of these costs are for billing transactions in our multi-payer system. Billing for an everyday primary care office visit consumes 13 minutes. In fact, the costs of billing activities for primary care physicians over a year amount to more than $99,000 per physician! [9]

4. "Ownership" of physicians as employees of hospitals, even insurers

Almost two-thirds of U. S. physicians are now employed by large employers, especially hospital systems and even by private insurers. Electronic health records (EHRs) have become billing instruments. Up-coding of the complexity of services is common, and physicians often don't know what is being charged for their services. That is determined by higher-up billing clerks and administrators.

Dr. Marni James-Carey, executive director of the Association of Independent Doctors, sums up the problem this way:

We know that when corporate medicine takes over the practice of independent medicine, costs go up, quality goes

down, and patients and doctors lose. This is all about cap-
turing market share so you can have more bargaining power
with payers, and get more money in reimbursement for the
same procedure. That's what causes prices to go up. [10]

5. Profiteering, even fraud.

Profiteering has become rampant across most parts of our
market-based system, as these examples show:

- Big PhRMA maximizes its profits in many ways,
  including direct-to-consumer advertising (banned in
  many countries), delaying competition from generics,
  non-rigorous "research" for marketing purposes,
  lobbying against negotiated drug prices and importation
  of drugs from other countries, and increasing drug prices
  to astronomical levels, such as the recent controversy
  over the emergency drug Epipen. The new gold-standard
  triple therapy for H.I.V. costs $39,000 a year in this
  country, compared to just $75 in Africa! [11]
- Overpayments to private Medicaid plans are endemic
  in more than 30 states, often involving unnecessary or
  duplicative payments to providers. [12]
- "Related party transactions" bring higher profits to three
  out of four of the nation's 11,000 nursing homes without
  being recorded in their financial records, and as they also
  cut nursing staff and put patients at increased risk. [13]

Fraud is also common in our under-regulated non-system.
Medical billing fraud has been estimated to account for about 10
percent of all health care costs, or about $270 billion a year. [14]

Miami-Linken, a mid-size Ohio-based distributor, sent 11 million doses of opioids (oxycodone and hydrocodone) to Mingo, a rural county in West Virginia with a population of just 25,000, further fueling the opioid crisis and bringing on litigation. [15]

Ways in Which Insured Americans Cannot Afford Essential Health Care

Health care has already priced itself beyond the budgets of much of our population. According to the 2018 Milliman Medical Index, the typical working American family of four covered by an average employer-sponsored preferred provider organization (PPO) plan now pays an average of $28,000 a year for health care, including insurance premiums, cost-sharing, and forgone wage increases (for the employer contribution). [16] The Kaiser Family Foundation has found that one-third of Americans between the age of 18 to 64 have themselves or a family member had problems paying their medical bills, including 57 percent if they are sick. As a result, 72 percent put off vacations or household purchases, 59 percent used up all or most of their savings, and 41 percent took an extra job or worked more hours. [17]

Here are some of the many financial crises that many millions of Americans confront every day in dealing with medical bills even when being insured.

Living paycheck to paycheck

Tristan Berger, 47, lives in Tucson, Arizona. He was born with spina bifida, for which he had 16 reconstructive surgeries on his feet since age 13. After a series of falls, he was too disabled to continue working. Despite having insurance coverage through his wife's job at Walmart, together with some income from the Social Security program, he is barely able to pay for necessary care, having to decide each month whether to pay a utility or medical bill. He spent $12,000 in 2017 on care not covered by his health insurance, plus the same amount in 2018. As he says. "There's no savings. We're part of that percentage of Americans that are one paycheck from being destitute." [18]

Financial impact of being hospitalized

Just having been hospitalized can have a major, ongoing impact on the financial security of individuals and their families. A study of the economic consequences of hospitalization recently found that 10 percent of people in their 50's who were hospitalized never went back to work while others scaled back their hours or took lower-paying jobs. Figure 5.1 shows the impact of hospitalizations on falling incomes. [19]

This is one patient's story that illustrates this point.

Yolanda Carrero was well insured by her day care employer, where she had worked for 14 years, when she was diagnosed with breast cancer in 2014. She also had short-term disability coverage. After a mastectomy, she had a complicated course with an infection and two more surgeries. When she was able to return to work three months later, she could no longer lift infants or sit on the floor with them. Fortunately, her employer moved her to a less taxing job and allowed her to work part-time, but this was a big financial hit. She couldn't afford the rent, but her adult son helped to make ends meet. As she says in retrospect, "that was a rough few years." [20]

FIGURE 5.1

AVERAGE INCOME DROP AFTER HOSPITALIZATION

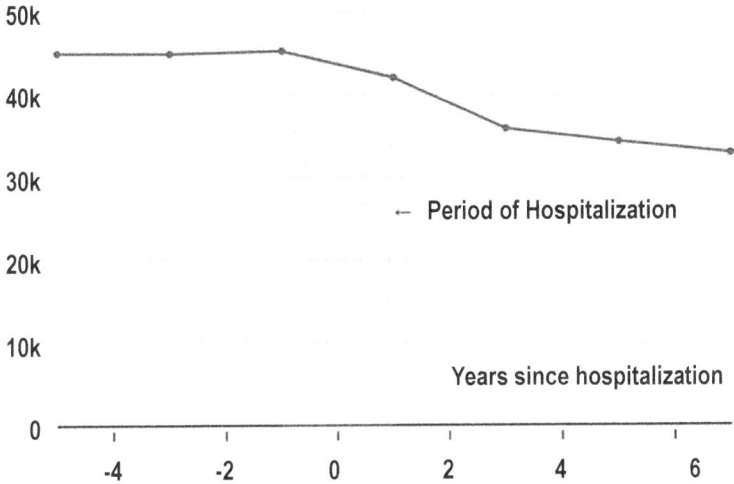

Source: Dobkin, C. et al, The Economic Consequences of Hospital Admissions.*The American Economic Review,* February, 2018

Surprise medical bills

According to a 2018 tracking poll by the Kaiser Family Foundation, four in ten adults say they had a surprise bill from a physician, hospital or laboratory over the past year. Figure 5.2 shows how worried recipients were about their ability to pay these bills. [21] These three patients' stories illustrate the problem.

When Drew Calver, 44, had a heart attack, he was hospitalized at St. David's Medical Center in Austin, Texas for four days, out of network for his insurer. His health plan paid almost $56,000, but the hospital charged him another $109,000, a so-called balance bill—the difference between *what the hospital and the insurer thought the care was worth. After Kaiser Health News and NPR published a story on this problem, Calver's bill was finally reduced to $332.* [22]

Roman Barshay, 46, a software engineer in Brooklyn, New York, took a bad fall when visiting friends in the Boston suburb of Chestnut Hill. He had trouble walking and had a sharp pain in his chest and back. An ambulance was called for the four-mile trip to a Boston hospital, for which he was later charged $3,360, or $915 for each mile, by Fallon Ambulance Service, a private company out of network for his insurer. The bill was sent to a collection agency, and Barshay reluctantly paid the bill.

Devin Hall, 67, a retired postal inspector in Northern California with stage 3 prostate cancer, is fighting a $7,109 bill from American Medical Response (AMR), the nation's largest ambulance provider. He developed rectal bleeding and was first taken to a hospital four miles away, but then referred to another hospital 20 miles away where he could receive specialist care. That hospital was in-network, but the ambulance was not. He was shocked to receive a bill from AMR for $8,460, for which the federal health plan, the Special Agents Mutual Benefit Plan, paid $1,350. Despite spending months on the phone calling the hospital, insurer, and AMR, the collection agency is still seeking the full balance of $7,109. [23]

FIGURE 5.2

HOW WORRIED ARE YOU ABOUT BEING ABLE TO AFFORD...
each of the following for you and your family?

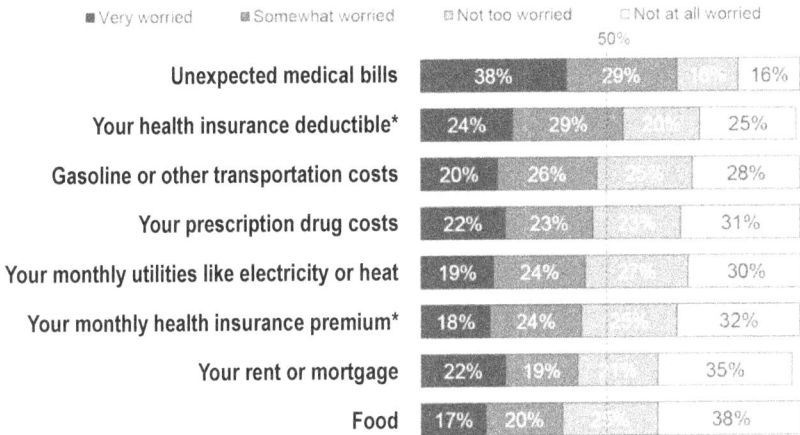

	Very worried	Somewhat worried	Not too worried	Not at all worried

				50%
Unexpected medical bills	38%	29%	16%	16%
Your health insurance deductible*	24%	29%	20%	25%
Gasoline or other transportation costs	20%	26%	25%	28%
Your prescription drug costs	22%	23%	23%	31%
Your monthly utilities like electricity or heat	19%	24%	27%	30%
Your monthly health insurance premium*	18%	24%	25%	32%
Your rent or mortgage	22%	19%	23%	35%
Food	17%	20%	25%	38%

Source: Kaiser Family Foundation, August 23-28, 2018, Peterson-Kaiser Health System Tracker.

Private collection agencies and health care costs

A 2018 report by the ACLU, *A Pound of Flesh: The Criminalization of Private Debt*, exposed a privatized web of injustices of scandalous proportions that pervades private collection agencies. Here are some of the findings of this report.

- One in three Americans have debts turned over to a private collection agency.
- Private debt collectors have entered into hundreds of partnerships with local district attorneys' offices to get people to pay on bounced check claims under threat of prosecution.
- Threatening letters are sent for bounced checks as low as $2.00.

- 90 percent of debt cases conclude in a default judgment against the defendant, with less than 2 percent of them represented by an attorney.
- Although debtors' prisons were banned in the U. S. more than 185 years ago, laws in 44 states and federal rules of civil and bankruptcy procedure expressly authorize debtors to be arrested and jailed for contempt of court.
- The victims of this under recognized scandal often struggle to recover from a lost job, mounting medical bills, death of a family member, divorce, illness, or are unable to work due to disabilities; black and Latino people are disproportionately affected.

Jennifer Turner, author of the ACLU report, sums up this unfair situation:

> *The private debt collection industry uses prosecutors and judges as weapons against millions of Americans who can't afford to pay their bills. Consumers have little chance of justice when our courts take the debt collector's side in almost every case—even to the point of ordering people jailed until they pay up. Courts are issuing arrest warrants and serving as taxpayer-funded tools of the multi-billion-dollar debt collection industry.* [24]

Unfortunately, this situation is now even worse as the Trump administration in early 2019 has taken steps to gut regulations from protecting families from predatory payday lenders. [25]

Annual and lifetime limits

The Trump administration has been offering waivers to states to put some kind of limits on Medicaid benefits, perhaps even including lifetime caps. Five states—Maine, Arizona, Utah, Wisconsin and Kansas— have already started this process of cutting back Medicaid benefits. Critics of this policy note that this would shift Medicaid from a health care safety net program for the poor and sick to a welfare program. [26] This patient's story illustrates the dire stakes involved if lifetime caps on coverage are imposed.

After my double mastectomy two years ago, I had to read two terrifying things: my pathology report and my hospital bill. The pathology report made me sink to the floor with despair; it noted multiple large tumors that had invaded my skin, and 15 underarm lymph nodes bursting with rapidly dividing cancer cells. I would require months of aggressive treatment.

The bill for my hospital stay and surgery was $173,000. But there was some good news: my insurance plan paid for all of it. For this, I thanked the Affordable Care Act, because it mandated that hospitalization—and everything else I needed, including lab tests, medication, and physical therapy—be covered as part of a set of essential benefits. My cumulative expenses now exceed $500,000, but the Affordable Care Act also bars insurance companies from putting a lifetime cap on what they will spend. So if my cancer returns, a real possibility since I'm 33 with poor prognostic factors, I won't have to choose between dying or going bankrupt. [27]

Seniors

Corporate stakeholders profiteer off the backs of U. S. seniors in multiple ways, often below the radar of public scrutiny. Here are two examples.

Big PhRMA

A 2018 report from the Committee on Homeland Security and Governmental Affairs examined the devastating effects of spiraling prices of prescription drugs on Medicare Part D beneficiaries. The 20 most prescribed drugs were looked at, including Crestor, Lyrica, Restasis, Symbicort, Tamiflu, and Xarelto. For 12 of the drugs, the prices went up by 50 percent between 2012 and 2017; for 6, the prices skyrocketed up by more than 100 percent over that period. The average annual change for the 20 drugs was an increase of 12 percent a year, about 10 times the average annual rate of inflation. [28]

Insurers

The airwaves are full of deceptive pitches urging seniors to enroll in a private Medicare Advantage plan, claiming that they will get more coverage than in traditional Medicare and that it will save them money compared to a Medigap supplemental plan. This has become a huge cash cow for Medicare Advantage insurers, who have various ways to game the system at taxpayers' expense. The six biggest Medicare Advantage companies—Aetna, Anthem, Centene, Cigna, Humana, and UnitedHealth (the largest)— game the system by fraudulently increasing the risk scores for severity of illness of their enrollees, thereby securing larger overpayments from the federal government. The Department of Justice is currently investigating this practice by all of these companies.

As these insurers have to pay out more for the care of these "sicker" enrollees, the patients commonly dis-enroll, typically citing overly restrictive network and less choice of physician and hospital. After dis-enrolling and returning to traditional Medicare, these patients often can't get a supplemental Medigap plan (that covers the 20 percent of costs not covered by Medicare), which they could have purchased if they had started with Medicare, not Medicare Advantage. [29]

The market for long-term care insurance has become increasingly unstable in recent years. This couple thought they had some security of coverage through their long-term care insurance plan until they found otherwise.

David and Sally Wylie, retired in their late 60s on Vinal-haven Island in Maine, had long-term care insurance for the last ten years. Over that period, the cost of their insurance through CNA Financial Corp. increased by more than 90 percent, putting a severe strain on their budget. [30]

Nursing home care

The costs of long-term care are way beyond the reach of most people in this country today. Two-thirds of U. S. nursing homes are for-profit, putting revenues before service. Private nursing home rooms now average more than $92,000 a year. [31] Medicare does not cover long-term stays; Medicaid can provide coverage only after patients spend down to eligible levels. This patient's story illustrates the fragility of nursing home care.

Maria Elena Flores, 64, was working as a home health aide for seniors near San Ysidro, California, when she had to give up that job to provide the same care for her husband when he was recovering from triple cardiac bypass surgery. His health then declined as he developed vascular dementia with erratic behavior that caused her to fall and injure her back. He was admitted to one nursing home but later discharged because of his behavior. The local hospital was unable to find another place for him, so Maria brought him back home under her care. [32]

Medical bankruptcy

Despite progress by the ACA in reducing the numbers of uninsured Americans, 84 million people are now underinsured, including many with employer-based insurance. A recent report tells us that Americans borrowed $88 billion in 2019 to cover their costs of health care. [33] A new study has found that two-thirds of personal bankruptcies, involving 530,000 families each year, are now caused by illness and medical bills. Dr. David Himmelstein, lead researcher and author of the study, summarized the problem this way:

Unless you're Bill Gates, you're just one serious illness away from bankruptcy. For middle-class Americans, health insurance offers little protection. Most of us have policies with so many loopholes, copayments, and deductibles that illness can put you in the poorhouse. And even the best job-based insurance often vanishes when prolonged illness causes job loss—just when families need it most. [34]

This couple's experience shows that affluent middle-class working Americans can get taken down to bankruptcy due to medical bills despite their best efforts to avoid it.

> *John and Carla Jordan in Stafford County, Virginia, had an Anthem Inc. insurance policy for the family through Carla's job as a public school teacher. Little more than ten years ago, their annual income was more than $100,000 through John's carpentry business and Carla's computer science teaching position in the local high school. But when John's business failed to recover after the housing boom and the Recession, and with Carla's salary virtually stable, a cascade of medical bills forced them to declare bankruptcy. They were facing huge bills for the care of John's seizures and a serious infection, together with Carla's diabetes and gallstone. Although the couple were still earning $79,000 before taxes in 2017, they were living paycheck-to-paycheck with no savings for their children to go to college or for their future retirement. Confronted by ever-increasing deductibles and mounting medical debts and collection agencies, they filed for bankruptcy a second time.* [35]

Conclusion

These examples show how unfair and cruel our current "system" is in supposedly the wealthiest nation in the world with huge costs of health care, even for those with insurance. The costs are increasingly unaffordable and propelled ever upward due to greed of corporate stakeholders and administrative waste in our profit-driven, unaccountable "system." These patient stories tell how important the stakes have become, and show clearly the need for the largest possible risk pool—universal coverage for our entire population—that will share the costs of illness and care.

We will return to this subject in Part III, but for now we turn to the next chapter to consider other ways in which the quality of our health care falls so far short of acceptable.

References:

1. Martin, AB, Hartman, M, Washington, B et al. National health care spending in 2017: Growth slows to post-great recession rates; share of GDP stabilizes. *Health Affairs*, December 6, 2018.

2. Papanicolas, I, Woskie, LR, Jha, AK. Health care spending in the United States and other high-income countries. *JAMA*, March 13, 2018.

3. Siegel, R, Columbus, C. As cost of U. S. health care skyrockets, so does pay of health care CEOs. *NPR*, July 26, 2017.

4. Scully, T. As quoted by Davidson, A. The President wants you to get rich on Obamacare. *New York Times Magazine*, October 13, 2013.

5. Commerce Dept. Service Annual Surveys and MedPac, 2016.

6. Fulton, BD. Health and market competition trends in the United States: Evidence and policy responses. *Health Affairs*, September 2017.

7. Abelson, R. When hospitals merge to save money, patients often pay more. *New York Times*, November 14, 2018.

8. Mathews, AW. Secret hospital deals drive rising health costs. *Wall Street Journal*, September 19, 2018: A1.

9. Tseng, P, Kaplan, RS, Richman, JD et al. Administrative costs associated with physician billing and insurance-related activities at an academic health care system. *JAMA*, February 20, 2018.

10. James-Carey, M. As quoted by Gamble, H. Is private equity helping or hurting healthcare? *Modern Healthcare*, July 10, 2018.

11. Rosenberb, T. H.I.V. drugs cost $75 in Africa, $39,000 in the U. S. Does it matter? *New York Times*, September 18, 2018.

12. Herman, B. Medicaid's unmanaged managed care. *Modern Healthcare*, April 30, 2016.

13. Rau, J. Care suffers as more nursing homes feed money into corporate webs. *Kaiser Health News*, December 31, 2017.

14. Buchheit, P. Private health care as an act of terrorism. *Common Dreams*, July 20, 2015, p. 1.

15. Bever, L. A town of 3,200 was flooded with nearly 21 million pain pills as addiction crisis worsened, lawmakers say. *The Washington Post*, January 31, 2018.

16. Girod, GS, Hart, SK, Weltz, SA. 2018 Milliman Medical Index. *Milliman Research Report*, May 21, 2018.

17. Altman, D. The medical bill score. How the public judges health care. *Axios*, October 3, 2017.

18. Sanger-Katz, M. 1,495 Americans describe the financial reality of being really sick. *New York Times*, October 17, 2018.

19. Dobkin C, Finklestein, A, Kluender, R et al.The economic consequences of hospital admissions. *The American Economic Review*, February, 2018.

20. Sanger-Kaatz, M. Getting sick can be really expensive, even for the insured. *New York Times*, March 21, 2018.

21. Altman, D. Surprise medical bills could be a powerful campaign issue. *Axios*, September 24, 2018.

22. Andrews, M, Appleby, J. The remedy for surprise medical bills may lie in stitching up federal law. *Kaiser Health News*, September 10, 2018.

23. Bailey, M. Taken for a ride? Ambulances stick patients with surprise bills. *Kaiser Health News*, November 27, 2017.

24. Turner, J. *A Pound of Flesh: The Criminalization of Private Debt.* American Civil Liberties Union Report, February 21, 2018.

25. Johnson, J. Siding with 'loan sharks' over consumers, Trump CFPB moves to gut payday lender regulations. *Common Dreams*, February 6, 2019.

26. Weixel, N. House Dems warn against Medicaid lifetime limits. *The Hill*, March 8, 2018.

27. Cohen, S. Breast cancer is political. Tie that up in your pink ribbon. *Los Angeles Times*, October 1, 2018.

28. Report details how skyrocketing prescription drug costs are harming nation's seniors. *Common Dreams*, March 26, 2018.

29. Rettino, J, Potter, W. How health insurers drive huge profits off of older Americans. *Tarbell*, October 11, 2018.

30. Scism, L. Safety net frays for millions of retirees. *Wall Street Journal*, January 18, 2018.

31. Associated Press. Study: Costs for most long-term care keep climbing. *New York Times*, May 10, 2018.

32. Ibid # 18, p. 4.

33. Higgins, E. 'Making money off dysfunction': Bolstering Medicare for All case, survey shows Americans accrued $88 billion in healthcare debt in 2018. *Common Dreams*, April 2, 2019.

34. Himmelstein, DU, Lawless, RM, Thorne, D et al. Medical bankruptcy: Still common despite the Affordable Care Act. *Am J Public Health*, March, 2019.

35. Tozzi, J, Tracer, Z. Sky-high deductibles broke the U. S. health insurance system. *Bloomberg*, June 26, 2018.

CHAPTER 6

"WITHOUT ACCESS, I HAVE NO QUALITY OF CARE"

The first five chapters of this book focused on how much of our population has poor and worsening access to health care, even for many with health insurance. Now we shift gears to look at ways that the quality of health care that Americans receive is unacceptable and much below what other countries with universal access to care receive.

This chapter has two goals: (1) to describe how a growing number of Americans forgo care because of unaffordable costs, then have worse outcomes later on if they ever do receive care; and (2) to consider the collision between costs, access and quality of future health care in this country as financially toxic new technological advances emerge.

How Access, Prices and Quality of Health Care Are Intertwined

It is an obvious but often disregarded fact that there can be no quality of care without good access to that care. Runaway prices in a profit-driven "system" have become a huge barrier to both access and quality of care in this country. As a result of trends described in the last chapter, here are examples of health care prices, as recently reported by the first annual report from Kaiser Health

News and NPR in their new investigation, 'Bill of the Month':

- Elizabeth Moreno's $18,000 urine test, purportedly to screen for opioids after surgery.
- Anne Soloviev's $1,500-a-month lotion for toenail fungus that didn't work.
- Benjamin Hynden's $9,000 CAT scan in an ER, despite having had a similar scan just a few weeks before for $268.
- Sherry Young's bill for minor foot surgery included more than $15,000 in charges for four small screws.
- Wren Veten's $92,000 bait-and-switch bill for gender confirmation surgery, though the price had been listed online for under $25,000.
- Drew Calver's $109,000 bill for out-of-network care of his heart attack.
- Dr. Naveed Khan's $56,000 bill for an air ambulance transport.
- Janet Winston's $48,000 bill for allergy skin testing.
- Shereese Hickson's bill for $123,000 for two new multiple sclerosis treatments, despite her being on both Medicare and Medicaid.
- Sarah Witter's $43,000 bill for two surgeries after a metal plate for her fractured leg from a skiing accident needed replacement. [1]

Unfortunately, these outlandish prices are not at all rare, and keep increasing through profiteering in a deregulated time under the Trump administration.

None of this is new, as Steven Brill found out several years ago. As an attorney and journalist, he was insured through Aetna, the third largest health insurer in the country. After receiving a bill for $197,000 after eight days in the hospital for treatment of an aortic aneurism, he met with Aetna's CEO trying to understand an explanation of benefits in his complex hospital bill. Together they could not do that, as described in his 2015 book, *America's Bitter Pill: Money, Politics, Backroom Deals, and the Fight to Fix Our Broken Healthcare System.* At the time, he observed that the ACA had failed to contain health care costs for these reasons:

> *It's about money: Healthcare is America's largest industry by far, employing one-sixth of the country's workforce. And it is the average American family's largest single expense, whether paid out of their pockets or through taxes and insurance premiums. . . In a country that treasures the marketplace. . . how much taming can we do when the healthcare industry spends four times as much on lobbying as the number two Beltway spender, the much-feared military-industrial complex.* [2]

Bringing all this down to family budgets, American households of four people, as was mentioned in the last chapter, now pay out an average of $28,000 a year for insurance and care, according to the 2018 Milliman Medical Index. [3] These high and unsustainable increases are not due to increase in services, but to *unimpeded price increases in a corporate-run market.* Figure 6.1 shows how prices and spending for health care have been increasing while the utilization of some, especially inpatient services, have been sharply declining. As Niall Brennan, CEO of the Health Care Cost Institute, observes: "The bottom line is, Americans are using less health care and paying more for it every year." [4]

FIGURE 6.1

CUMULATIVE CHANGE IN HEALTH CARE PRICES, USE, AND SPENDING, 2012 - 2016

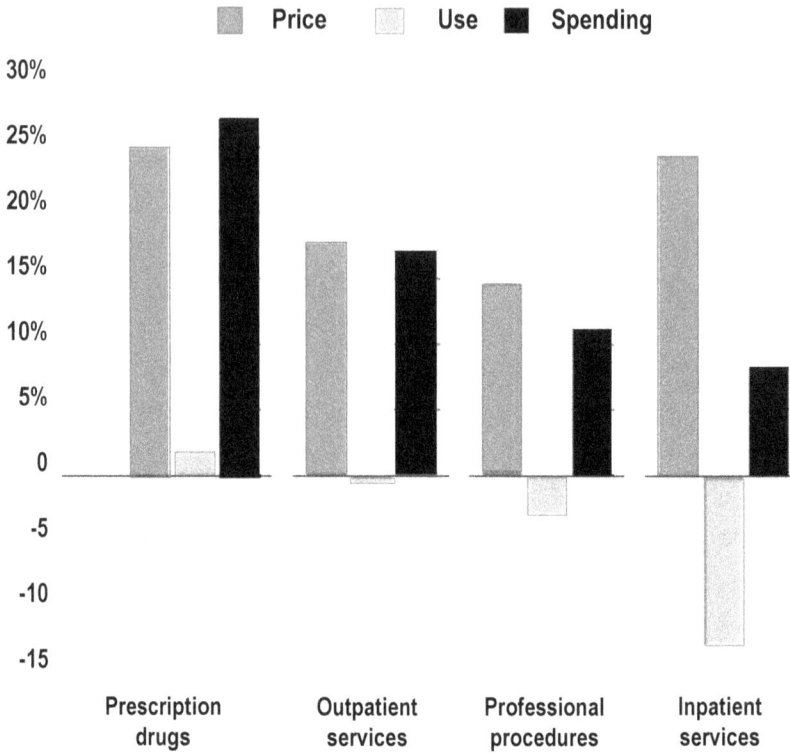

■ Price ☐ Use ■ Spending

30%

25%

20%

15%

10%

5%

0

-5

-10

-15

| Prescription drugs | Outpatient services | Professional procedures | Inpatient services |

Source: Health Care Cost Institute.

Here is an extreme example of how some Americans feel disengaged from *any* health care because of unaffordable costs.

When a woman became trapped between a subway car and platform in Boston, she pleaded with bystanders not to help her, saying that she couldn't afford either an ambulance or hospital care. Weeping and in agony, she finally accepted help and an ambulance after EMTs arrived. [5]

Delaying or forgoing essential health care because of unaffordable costs has increasingly become the norm in the United States. According to the Peterson-Kaiser Health System Tracker, one in ten adults either delayed or did not receive medical care due to cost in 2016. A recent study found that women who were switched to high deductible employer-based insurance experienced delays of five to seven months in diagnosis of early-stage breast cancer, likely associated with worse outcomes. [6]

Figure 6.2 breaks these numbers down by type of health care service. [7]

FIGURE 6.2

PERCENT OF ADULTS WHO REPORT DELAYING AND/OR GOING WITHOUT MEDICAL CARE DUE TO COSTS, BY TYPE OF CARE, 2016

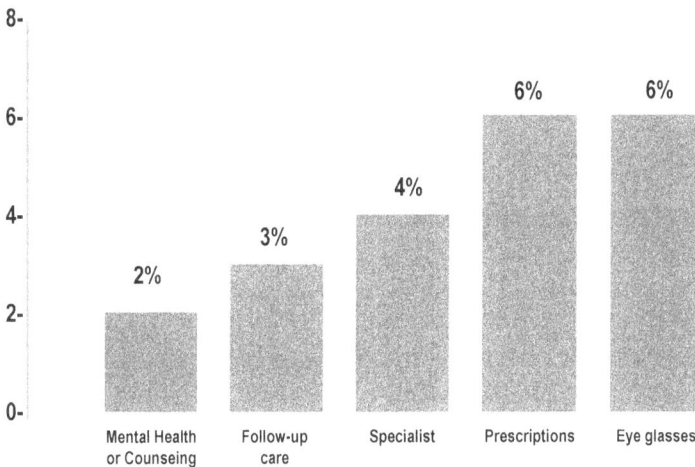

Source: Kaiser Family Foundation analysis of National Health Interview Survey.

The *2017 Commonwealth Fund International Health Policy Survey of Older Adults* found that U. S. seniors are sicker than their counterparts in ten other high-income countries as they face greater financial barriers to care, even in spite of their having universal access available through traditional Medicare. More than one-third of U. S. seniors report having three or more chronic conditions, and struggle to deal with high costs of care as "high need" patients. Almost one-third of these chronically ill patients skip care because of costs, compared to just 2 percent in Sweden. [8] Moreover, a recent study found that socioeconomically vulnerable Canadians are consistently and highly advantaged on health care access and outcomes compared to their American counterparts, and that we can expect that more than 50 million Americans will die earlier over the next generation unless the U. S. moves to a system of universal coverage. [9]

These are some common situations where patients of all ages have to forgo or delay care at the time of need due to the high costs of that care.

Immediate cash shortages

A recent study found that many people make decisions about when to receive and pay for health care based on whether they have cash on hand. This pattern is not seen just in lower-income people, but can cause those with higher incomes to delay care in the context of increasing out-of-pocket health care spending. One in six families makes an extraordinary payment of $2,000 in a single month for health care, stressing liquid assets and leading to higher credit card debt. Health care spending is also closely related to other factors, such as job loss, natural disasters, and mortgage rate changes. Although conservatives tell us that health savings accounts can effectively address this problem, most people cannot afford to invest in them, and if they do, there is not enough money there when they need it. [10]

Unaffordable copayments

> *Heather Holland, 38, a second grade teacher, fell sick*
> *with the flu and planned to pick up medication. But she felt*
> *the co-payment of $116 was too high. When her husband,*
> *Frank, found this out, he bought the prescription himself, but*
> *she soon became much worse. She ended up being hospital-*
> *ized in an ICU and receiving dialysis, but died two days later*
> *due to complications of the flu, leaving behind her husband*
> *and two children ages 7 and 10.* [11]

Unaffordable prescription drugs

As we saw in the last chapter, the costs of the most commonly prescribed brand-name drugs have gone up at a rate about 10 times the inflation rate over the last five-year period. As a result, a 2015 report from the CDC found that about 25 million people did not take their medication as prescribed, either skipping doses or not refilling prescriptions. [12] At the same time shifting to generic drugs doesn't help consumers much. Going generic often does not lower their prices, and frequently increases them. As just one example, a 2015-2016 data analysis of Medicaid drug costs by *Kaiser Health News* found that the price of the original branded pain-killer Aleve as a generic went up by 136 percent over that year, costing Medicaid an additional $10 million. [13]

Future U. S. Health Care: Collision Between What's Possible but Inaccessible

The overwhelming costs of new, cutting edge treatments raise serious, not yet asked or answered questions about what patients, taxpayers, and society can afford as technical advances break beyond today's price and cost barriers. These questions are certain to have enormous economic implications and can be expected to also raise moral questions about who deserves these treatments, who should decide, and whether their cost-benefits are acceptable for governments at all levels and for society overall.

Here are two examples that threaten to break the bank.

Organ transplants

Almost all of the 250 transplant centers across the country require patients to verify how they will cover bills that can total $400,000 for a kidney transplant or $1.3 million for a heart transplant, plus an average of $2,500 a month for anti-rejection drugs that must be taken for life. These are average costs for some transplants in 2017, including pre-and post-op costs and immunosuppressant drugs:

Heart-lung	$2,564,000
Kidney-heart	$2,530,900
Heart	$1,382,400
Liver	$812,500

Patients needing transplants are typically denied surgery and care unless and until they are able to raise large amounts of money. They all receive a "wallet biopsy." They are expected to approach such fund-raising options as GoFundMe or HelpHopeLive to raise the necessary funds. Transplant centers refer potential patients to a single national registry. More than 114,000 people are now on the waiting list for organs in the U. S., with fewer than 35,000 organs having been transplanted in 2017.

This patient's story illustrates the obstacles faced by patients needing transplant surgery.

Hedda Martin, 60, of Grand Rapids, Michigan, was denied a heart transplant because of inability to pay for it. She was told to start a fundraising effort with an initial goal of $10,000. She was able to raise more than $30,000 through social media and a GoFundMe account, which was enough to at least put her on the national waiting list. [14]

Precision medicine

Kristen Kilmer, 38, was diagnosed with incurable breast cancer in 2015. She had lost her own mother as a teenager, and was hoping to get more time to be with her 8-year-old daughter. She searched for experimental treatments, opting for an unproven approach whereby researchers select treatments based on the unique, ever-changing DNA of her cancer cells. In 2018, at 41, she has done better than she might have expected, with her tumors no longer visible on scans, but her prognosis is still very much guarded.

Kristen's insurance company calls her treatments experimental, covering only a fraction of her care. She has been forced to stop taking a drug costing $17,000 a month (Lynparza, manufactured by AstraZeneca) or burdening her family with a huge debt. Financial assistance was provided by the manufacturer for much of the first three years on the drug, but that assistance has recently been stopped. Another way patients can receive assistance is by enrolling in a clinical trial, which can provide drugs for free, but that still requires patients to get to such trial centers. For Kristen, that involves a 12-hour round trip drive every month to Sioux Falls, South Dakota.

Over the last three years, Kristen has spent about $80,600 out-of-pocket treating her illness. She is still up against the basic dilemma she started with—whether or not to continue her treatment and not wanting to put her family in a mountain of debt. [13]

Looking to the future, we have to realize that patients, families, and society cannot possibly afford these kinds of advanced treatments for everyone who needs them as long as we have a for-profit multi-payer financing system with segmented risk pools that serve private insurers more than the common good.

Conclusion

We will return to some of these issues in Part III, but now we need to go to the next chapter where we will consider ways other than unaffordable costs that threaten and lower the quality of care being received by Americans in a "system" that favors revenue seeking by corporate stakeholders more than the needs of patients, families, and taxpayers.

References:

1. Year one of KHN's 'Bill of the Month': A kaleidoscope of financial challenges. *Kaiser Health News*, December 21, 2018.
2. Brill, S. *America's Bitter Pill: Money, Politics, Backroom Deals, and the Fight to Fix Our Broken Healthcare System.* New York. *Random House,* 2015, pp. 7-8.
3. Milliman Medical Index, 2018.
4. Mathews, AW. New tactics on health costs. *Wall Street Journal*, December 4, 2018, R10.

5. Conley, J. 'I can't afford that': Trapped and injured by subway car, woman begged bystanders not to call ambulance due to expense. *Common Dreams*, July 4, 2018.
6. Wharam, JF, Zhang, F, Wallace, J et al. Vulnerable and less vulnerable women in high-deductible health plans experience delayed breast cancer care. *Health Affairs*, March 2019.
7. Cox, C, Sawyer, B. How does cost affect access to care? Peterson-Kaiser Health System Tracker. *Kaiser Family Foundation*, 2016.
8. Osborn, R, Doty, MM, Moulds, D et al. Older Americans were sicker and faced more financial barriers to health care than counterparts in other countries. 2017 Commonwealth Fund International Health Policy Survey of Older Adults, November 15, 2017. New York. *Commonwealth Fund.*
9. Escobar, KM, Murariu, D, Munro, S. Care of acute conditions and chronic diseases in Canada and the United States: Rapid systematic review and meta-analysis. *Journal of Public Health Research*, March 11, 2019.
10. Farrell, D, Greig, F, Hamoudi, A et al. Cash flow dynamics and family health care spending: Evidence from banking data. Health Policy Brief. *Health Affairs*, December 13, 2018.
11. Coyne, C, Gibson, J. Weatherford teacher dies from flu effects. *Weatherford Democrat*, February 5, 2018.
12. Report details how skyrocketing prescription drug costs are harming nation's seniors. *Common Dreams*, March 26, 2018.
13. Lupkin, S. Climbing costs of decades-old drugs threatens to break Medicaid bank. *Kaiser Health News*, August 14, 2017.
14. Aleccia, JN. No cash, no heart. Transplant centers require proof of payment. *Kaiser Health News*, December 5, 2018.
15. Szabo, L. Pricey precision medicine often financially toxic for cancer patients. *Kaiser Health News*, November 1, 2018.

CHAPTER 7

"MY CARE, WHEN I CAN GET IT, IS FRAGMENTED AND MIXED UP"

As we saw in the last chapter, unaffordable costs of health care lead many millions of Americans to delay or forgo care with later worse outcomes, if and when they finally do get care. There are also other important factors that put U. S. health care at or near the bottom compared with other high-income countries around the world.

This chapter has two goals: (1) to discuss six factors that fragment U. S. health care; and (2) to describe the poor and unacceptable quality of care that results from this chaotic non-system.

Fragmentation of U. S. Health Care
Inadequate primary care

Primary care by definition includes *all* of these four basic features: (1) first-contact care; (2) longitudinal continuity of care over time; (3) comprehensiveness, with capacity to manage the majority of health problems for which patients seek care; and (4) coordination of care with other parts of the health care system. [1] Some specialties can deal with some of these functions, such as emergency medicine physicians for first-contact care or opthalmologists providing continuity of eye care over years, but they are not providing primary care.

Given the absence of a national physician workforce plan concerned with the goal to produce a solid proportion of U. S. medical school graduates entering primary care residencies and practice, we have had a long-standing shortage of primary care physicians in this country. The proportion of generalist physicians declined from 43 percent in 1965 to less than 30 percent in 1990, when only 11.5 percent were in general or family practice. [2]

Today, fewer than 10 percent of U. S. medical school graduates opt for family practice. Some internists become primary care physicians for adults and children, but most of their colleagues leave primary care for subspecialties. Most U. S. medical graduates enter the highly reimbursed specialties of radiology, orthopedic surgery, anesthesiology, and dermatology (ROAD). The nation is now facing a shortage of 52,000 primary care physicians by 2025. [3] Due in large part to higher reimbursement of procedural and non-primary care services, we are also facing shortages of other time-intensive specialties, especially geriatrics and psychiatry.

Between 2005 and 2015, disproportionate losses took place in primary care physician supply, decreasing from 46.6 to 41.4 per 100,000 population, with greater losses in rural areas. That study also found that every increase of 10 primary care physicians per 100,000 population was associated with reduced cardiovascular, cancer, and respiratory mortality by 0.9 % to 1.4 %. [4]

As a result of the primary care shortage, many patients with acute or chronic medical problems have a hard time seeing a physician, instead receiving inadequate care through emergency rooms without adequate follow-up or preventive care, especially involving underserved minority populations. In her 2018 book, *Becoming*, Michelle Obama, who grew up in South Chicago, describes how inadequate health care was there in 2002 when she worked at the University of Chicago Medical Center as executive director for community affairs.

> *The south side [of Chicago] has just over a million res-*
> *idents and a dearth of medical providers, not to mention a*
> *population that was disproportionately affected by the kinds*
> *of chronic conditions that tend to afflict the poor—asthma,*
> *diabetes, hypertension, heart disease. With huge numbers*
> *of people uninsured and many others dependent on Med-*
> *icaid, patients regularly jammed the university hospital's*
> *emergency room, often seeking what amounted to routine*
> *nonemergency treatment or having gone on so long without*
> *preventive care that they were now in dire need of help. The*
> *problem was glaring, expensive, inefficient, and stressful for*
> *everyone involved. ER visits did little to improve anyone's*
> *long-term health, either.* [5]

According to the Peterson-Kaiser Health System Tracker, almost one-half of U. S. adults without health insurance in 2016 had no usual source of care (Figure 7.1), with two-thirds without a usual source of care going without preventive care (Figure 7.2).

As a result of the vacuum in primary care and the near-disappearance of solo and small group practice, it has become exceptional for a patient and family to have and keep a primary care physician who knows them. More than 60 percent of U. S. physicians are now employed by others, especially by expanding hospital systems, where they are under the thumb of administrators to maximize revenue from their services. Clinical autonomy of physicians has suffered under this pervasive trend as their bureaucratic tasks have increased and are leading many to burnout and earlier retirement than planned.

FIGURE 7.1

PERCENT OF ADULTS WITHOUT A USUAL SOURCE OF CARE, BY HEALTH AND INSURANCE STATUS, 2016

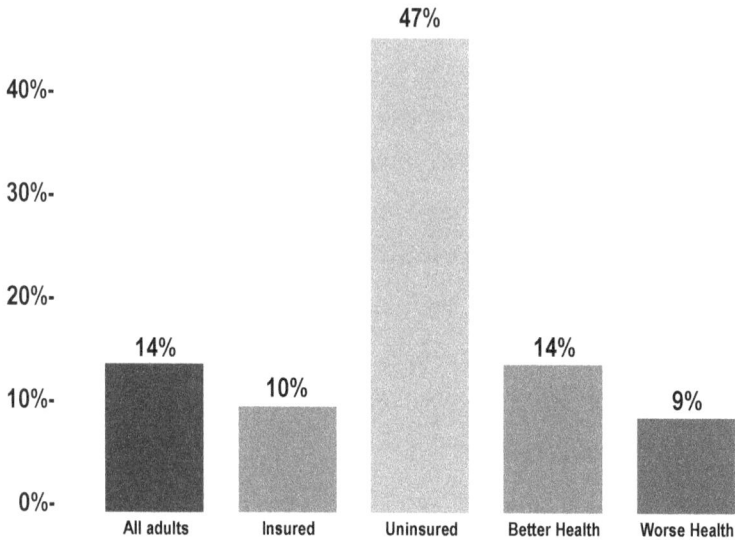

Source: Kaiser Family Foundation analysis of National Health Interview Survey. Peterson-Kaiser Health System Tracker.

As primary care has become less accessible for patients across the country, it has been largely replaced by a proliferation of urgent care centers for first-contact care, typically staffed by nurse practitioners and physician assistants, but without comprehensiveness, coordination, or continuity of care. Many patients, especially younger, healthier people, have given up on the idea of having a primary care physician, as this young man decided:

FIGURE 7.2

UNINSURED ADULTS WHO LACK A USUAL SOURCE OF CARE ARE ALSO MORE LIKELY TO FORGO PREVENTIVE CARE

Percent of adults without a usual source of care who reported
going without preventive care, 2016

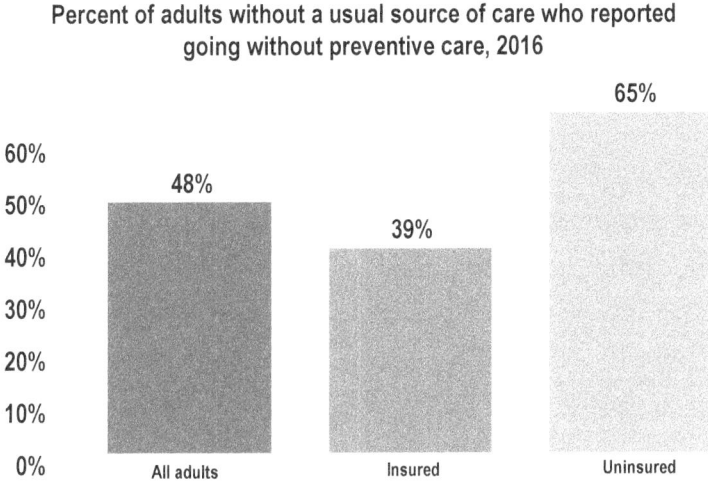

Source: Kaiser Family Foundation analysis of National Health Interview Survey. Peterson-Kaiser Health System Tracker.

Calvin Brown, 23, doesn't have a primary care physician, and doesn't want one. Since graduation from the University of San Diego in 2017, he has taken a series of jobs in several California cities. As a young person in a nomadic state, he prefers going to a walk-in clinic whenever he gets some illness. He sees himself as part of a new generation that sees health care as different from the traditional way of going to a primary care physician over years. As he says, "The whole 'going to the doctor' phenomenon is something that's fading from our generation. It means getting in a car [and] going to a waiting room." Instead, an urgent care visit costs him about $40 a visit and is more convenient—"like speed dating. Services are rendered in a quick manner." [6]

Lack of coordination of care

Too much of health care today involves patients being bounced around among non-primary care physicians, whether as outpatients or in hospitals. Lack of coordination within our increasingly fragmented, over-specialized health care non-system leads to worse quality of care, as this 2010 Report from the Josiah Macy, Jr. Foundation described well:

> *Too often, patients with acute or chronic health conditions receive services from multiple health providers in multiple care settings that do not coordinate and communicate with each other. This is especially true for the vulnerable elderly and disabled populations. This lack of coordination and integration leads to a fragmented health care system in which patients experience questionable care with more errors, more waste and duplication, and little accountability for quality and cost efficiency.* [7]

Communication problems

It was hoped that electronic health records (EHRs), as widely adopted in recent years, could improve communication, efficiency, patient safety, reduce duplicative services, and even save money. None of this has happened. EHRs have become billing instruments that tempt providers (and their employers) to up-code for higher reimbursement, thereby *raising* costs. Competing EHR systems generally don't talk to each other, and they are customized to each hospital that adopts them. Much of the "information" in their templates is irrelevant, and the patient's personal narrative is nowhere to be found. [8] As physicians (who increasingly need scribes during a patient visit) concentrate more on the EHR than looking at and talking with the patient, the doctor-patient relationship is intruded upon, thereby degrading the quality of clinical documentation and care. [9]

Primary care physicians who refer their patients for hospital care typically no longer see them in the hospital, where hospitalists try to serve as coordinators of inpatient care. But they generally don't know the patient's story, have never seen them before, don't communicate with the referring physician and often not adequately with other hospitalists on later shifts. Communication is also frequently inadequate between and among consulting specialists when they are called upon to care for one or another of the patient's multiple problems.

Decreased continuity of care

Continuity of care over years with a primary care physician has been at the core of the doctor-patient relationship for many years, but today is often a thing of the past. Under the guise of "competition" or "efficiency," that continuity has been lost. This trend has been accelerated by mergers and consolidation among hospital systems, business decisions of insurers, changing and more restricted networks, and instability created by accountable care organizations (ACOs).

One example of this disruptive trend was the receipt of certified letters sent to hundreds of patients at the University of Pittsburgh Medical Center (UPMC) in 2013 informing them that they could no longer see their physicians after their insurer had become both a rival hospital system and an insurer. Cancer patients in the middle of treatment were even cut off from their UPMC physicians. [10] Another disruptive trend occurs after hospitals buy up primary care physician practices, then keep future referrals for specialized services in-house without regard to patients' previous referral patterns. [11]

Unnecessary, inappropriate care

We have known for years that up to one-third of all health services provided in the U. S. are either unnecessary or inappropriate. [12] According to a 2016 national survey by the American Board of Internal Medicine, three of four physicians surveyed believe that unnecessary tests and procedures are a serious problem. [13] Here are three other markers of over-utilization of health care, especially related to our fragmented, profit-driven system:

- Polypharmacy is a common problem among older adults who see multiple physicians, who do not talk to one another, for chronic problems. [14]
- The overuse of elective cardiac catheterization, which carries significant risk. [15]
- Up to one-third of patients who undergo knee replacement continue to have chronic pain, with one in five dissatisfied with the results. [16]

Churning insurance coverage, even if still insured

As we saw in Chapter 3, the GOP and Trump administration have sabotaged many patient protections of the ACA even though they have failed to repeal it. We are already seeing divided health insurance markets where younger, healthier people purchase lightly regulated skinny plans with poor coverage while older sicker people face much higher costs for any kind of comprehensive coverage within an unstable, ever-changing marketplace that serves the needs of insurers, not patients. As more states seek federal waivers that allow them greater control of their markets, we can expect the burden on patients to increase. [17]

Here is just one example of the turmoil encountered by a physician as a patient in a supposedly progressive state, California, despite his expertise as a health policy expert.

> *Dr. Don McCanne, 81, retired family physician after 30 years of practice in San Clemente, California, called his primary care physician for a 90-day refill of his two blood pressure medications. His physician had recently retired and his practice was taken over by another physician. Don soon found himself dealing with OptumCare Medical Group, a subsidiary of UnitedHealth, and further learned through their website that he was assigned, without his knowledge, to their Medicare Pioneer ACO. After countless phone calls and long delays to an always-busy telephone system and non-responsive attempts to contact their website, these medications were finally issued, with errors and for only a 30-day supply. His local pharmacist of long standing was only authorized to refill 30-day requests; only Anthem's pharmacy benefit manager could provide 90-day renews, thus cutting out the business of the local pharmacy. Since then, Don and his wife left OptumCare, transferred their care to another physician, and signed up for a Medigap supplement to protect them from catastrophic events. [18]*

Poor Quality of Care in our Fragmented System
1. Depersonalization

As primary care in its full breadth continues to be unavailable to much of our population, first-contact care spreads out to many providers, facilities, and virtual facsimiles thereof. Examples include emergency rooms, urgent care clinics, "retail clinics" in shopping malls for walk-in care, long-distance call centers, and expanding use of telemedicine companies that offer virtual visits with physicians or other providers that never see, examine, or talk with the patient. Long gone from this mix is the traditional generalist family physician who gets to know patients and their narratives over years, often having made house calls and met other family members in their own environments.

Today's fragmented "system" depersonalizes patients as providers know little about each patient's story. This distancing that so frequently substitutes for first-contact care carries its own harms to quality of care, as these two examples illustrate:

- Hundreds of long-distance call centers have been established across the country in recent years. They are typically funded by insurers and housed in warehouse-like buildings with row upon row of small cubicles. Operators with little or no medical training work by protocol, often without access to nurses, as they respond to patients' questions around the clock. Operators are rewarded with bonuses if they limit visits to physicians or hospitals. Anthem even gave them bonuses up to 25 percent of their salaries if they met utilization targets for these services. [19]

- A 2016 study by researchers posing as patients with skin problems sought help from 16 online telemedicine companies. Key questions were not asked, diagnoses such as syphilis, herpes, and skin cancer were often misdiagnosed, and some of the on-line physicians were not licensed to practice where the patients lived. [20]

2. Insurance coverage matters

As health insurance markets further destabilize under the Trump administration, with loss of the ACA's patient protections, quality of care is harmed even for those who are insured. These are markers of this problem:

- Many policies being marketed today have poor benefits, such as minimal or no coverage of specialty drugs that may force cancer patients to forgo recommended treatment.
- Privatized Medicare plans tend to have worse patient outcomes than traditional Medicare, especially for sicker patients. [21]
- Privatized Medicaid plans also have worse outcomes than their public counterparts. [22]
- It has been estimated that 7,115 to 17,104 unnecessary deaths would occur attributable to the refusal of 20 states to expand Medicaid under the ACA after 2010. [23]

3. Worse outcomes due to increasing inequality and disparities

Inequality within the U. S. population has been steadily increasing in recent years to a point way beyond any sense of fairness. In this land of supposed plenty, there are 43 million Americans living in poverty out of our population of 326 million. [24] Almost two-thirds of tax cuts from the GOP's 2017 tax bill go to those with the top 20 percent of incomes, with the top 1 percent getting 83 percent of the gains. [25] In 1980, the top 1 percent took in 27 times more income than the bottom 50 percent; that multiple today has risen to at least 80. [26]

The growing part of our population with limited incomes and declining access to care is increasingly vulnerable to worse outcomes, including premature, preventable deaths. Dr. David Ansell, former chief of general medicine at Cook County Hospital in Chicago and author of the excellent 2017 book, *The Death Gap: How Inequality Kills*, observes:

> *Our current multi-payer for-profit health insurance system perpetuates premature death by putting many people at an extreme disadvantage when it comes to affording care. Those who have better health insurance policies can access better care. However, even patients with insurance cards face skyrocketing copays, deductibles and pharmaceutical prices that keep them from seeking care. Last year, 27 percent of Americans said they had postponed or avoided getting care they needed because of the cost; 23 percent said they had skipped a recommended test or treatment due to cost; and 21 percent said they had chosen not to fill prescriptions for medication because they couldn't afford it. . . . Death rates tell the same story. Since 1980, there have been dramatic gains in life expectancy for the top 20 percent of U. S. earners. At the same time, the poorest 20 percent have seen their life expectancy plummet. [27]*

Disparities in health care are also increasing in our profit-driven dysfunctional non-system. These disparities can be based on such factors as race/ethnicity, socioeconomic status, age, gender, location, and disability status. As one example among seniors, a recent study in New York State found that those hospitalized with private Medicare Advantage did worse than those with traditional Medicare, with black patients receiving worse post-hospital care resulting in higher readmission rates. [28] Giving out more state waivers, as the Trump administration is doing, will further increase disparities as state eligibility requirements become even more restrictive. In Alabama, as an example, one with an annual income above 18 percent of the federal poverty level (about $312 per month) is not eligible for Medicaid. [29]

4. Failure of 'pay-for-performance' to improve quality of care and save costs

What has been tried to reverse these trends in the U. S.? It's an interesting story over the last two decades, and we are still continuing failed policies aimed to decrease the costs of health care and improve its quality. 'Pay-for-performance' (P4P) has been a key concept of these policies that are intended to change how payments for health care are made by Medicare in an attempt to limit the volume of services in favor of their quality.

The first iteration of P4P, established by Medicare as the Value-Based Payment Modifier program, was succeeded in 2017 by a very similar program, the Merit-Based Incentive Payment System (MIPS). Both of these programs have offered bonuses to the top-performing physicians and practices, with penalties for practices that performed the worst. "Quality measures" are used, such as how often patients were hospitalized for preventable conditions, how often hospitalized patients were re-admitted to the hospital within a month of discharge, annual rates of mortality, and total Medicare spending per patient.

Despite the hype for P4P by policymakers, a 2017 study by researchers at Harvard Medical School and the University of Pittsburgh Graduate School of Public Health found that [the first P4P program] "failed to deliver on its central promise to increase value of care for patients. The program may have also exacerbated health disparities by inadvertently shifting payments from physicians caring for sicker, poorer patients to those caring for healthier, richer ones." [30]

Most physicians find P4P's "quality measures" frustrating and of doubtful clinical value. Some physicians worry that this approach will lead to pressures to avoid older and sicker patients. [31] In fact, that is happening since these "quality measures" are flawed by not accounting for socio-economic determinants of patient populations, leading to inappropriate penalties on safety net hospitals and physicians practicing in poorer and disadvantaged communities. [32]

There is now abundant evidence that P4P programs are a failure and should be abandoned. In a recent article, Drs. Sullivan (an attorney) and Soumerai (a professor of population medicine at Harvard Medical School) summarize the research that demonstrate how P4P policies penalize physicians:

- *Do not improve the health of patients.*
- *Harm sicker and poorer patients.*
- *Encourage doctors and hospitals to avoid or "fire" sicker patients who drag down quality scores due to factors outside physicians' control.*
- *Cause some doctors to stop using lifesaving treatments if they don't result in bonuses.*
- *Create interruptions in needed medical care.*
- *Reduce job satisfaction and undermine altruism and professionalism among doctors.* [33]

Conclusion

The last two chapters have shown how embedded poor and unacceptable quality of health care has become in the United States, despite the unfounded claims of some that it is the best in the world. Should government play a larger role in enabling Americans to have access to affordable care of good quality? Logical as that may sound, let's move to the next chapter to see how much oversight we are getting.

References

1. Starfield, B. Is primary care essential? *The Lancet* 344 (8930): 1129-1133, 1994.

2. Schroeder, SA. The troubled profession: Is medicine's glass half-full or half-empty? *Ann Intern Med* 116: 583-592, 1992.

3. Peterson, SM, Liaw, WR, Phillips, RL et al. Projecting U. S. primary care physician workforce needs: 2010-2025. *Ann Fam Med* 10 (6): 503-509, 2012.

4. Basu, S, Berkowitz, SA, Phillips, RL et al. Association of primary care physician supply with population mortality in the United States, 2005-2015. *JAMA* InternMed online, February 18, 2019.

5. Obama, M. *Becoming.* New York. *Crown*, p. 210.

6. Boodman, SG. Spurred by convenience, millennials often spurn the 'family doctor' model. *Kaiser Health News*, October 9, 2018.

7. Mitchener, JL, Berkowitz, B, Aguilar-Gaaxiola, S et al. Designing new models of care for diverse populations: Why new modes of care delivery are needed. In Cronenwett, L, Dzau, V, Cullitin, B, Russell, S (eds). *Who Will Provide Primary Care and How Will They Be Trained?* Proceedings of a conference sponsored by the Josiah Macy Jr. Foundation, Durham, NC 2010, pp. 84-85.

8. Abelson, R, Creswell, J, Palmer, G. Medicare bills rise as records turn electronic. *New York Times*, September 21, 2014.

9. Friedberg, MW, Chen, PG, Van Busum, KR et al. RAND Health Research Report. *Factors Affecting Physician Personal Satisfaction and Their Implications for Patient Care, Health Systems, and Health Policy.* Santa Monica, CA. *RAND Corporation*, 2013.

10. Brown, T. Out of network, out of luck. *New York Times*, October 15, 2013.

11. Mathews, AW, Evans, M. Hospitals push doctors to keep referrals in house. *Wall Street Journal*, December 28, 2018.

12 Wenner, JB, Fisher, ES, Skinner, JS. Geography and the debate over Medicare reform. *Health Affairs Web Exclusive*, W-103, February 13, 2002.

13. Hancock, J. How tiny are benefits from many tests and pills? Researchers paint a picture. *Kaiser Health News*, October 12, 2016.

14. Landro, L. Medication overload. *Wall Street Journal*, October 1, 2016: D1.

15. Patel, MR, Peterson, ED, Dai, MS et al. Low diagnostic yield of elective cardiac angiography. *N Engl J Med* 362: 862-895, 210.

16. Szabo, L. Up to a third of knee replacements pack pain and regret. *Kaiser Health News*, December 25, 2018.

17. Sanger-Katz, M. A big divergence is coming in health care among states. *New York Times*, February 18, 2018.

18. McCanne, D. I just want my blood pressure pills, dammit! Quote of the Day, September 17, 2018. don@mccanne.org

19. Bartlett, DL, Steele, JB. *Critical Condition: How Health Care in America Became Big Business & Bad Medicine.* New York. *Doubleday*, 2004: pp. 182-189.

20. Beck, M. Websites misdiagnose ailments. *Wall Street Journal*, May 16, 2016: A6.

21. Gold, M, Casillas, G. What do we know about health care access and quality in Medicare Advantage versus the traditional Medicare program? *Kaiser Family Foundation*, November 6, 2014.

22. McCue, MJ, Bailit, MH. Assessing the financial health of Medicaid managed care plans and the quality of care they provide. New York. *The Commonwealth Fund*, June 15, 2011.

23. Dickman, S et al. Opting out of Medicaid expansion: The health and financial impacts. *Health Affairs Blog*, January 30, 2014.

24. Powers, N. Fear of a black planet: Under the Republican push for welfare cuts, racism boils. *Truthout*, January 21, 2018.

25. Matthews, D. The Republican tax bill got worse: Now the top 1% gets 83% of the gains. *Vox*, December 18, 2017.

26. Boushey, H. The tax bill should've been called the Inequality Exacerbation Act of 2017. *The Hill*, December 22, 2017.

27. Ansell, D. I watched my patients die of poverty for 40 years. It's time for single payer. *The Washington Post*, September 13, 2017.

28. Li, Y, Cen, X, Thirukamaran, CP et al. Medicare Advantage associated with more racial disparity than traditional Medicare for hospital readmissions. *Health Affairs*, July 2017.

29. Cunningham, PW. Here are three big ways the Trump administration could put its mark on Medicaid. *The Washington Post*, May 16, 2018.

30. Roberts, ET, Zaslavsky, J, McWilliams, JM. The Value-Based Payment Modifier: Program outcomes and implications for disparities. *Ann Intern Med* on line, November 28, 2017.

31. Mathews, AW. Hospitals prescribe big data to track doctors at work. *Wall Street Journal*, July 11, 2013: A1.

32. Ryan, J, Doty, MM, Hamel, L et al. Primary care providers' views of recent trends in health care delivery and payment. *The Commonwealth Fund and the Kaiser Family Foundation*, August 5, 2015.

33. Sullivan, K, Soumerai, S. Pay for performance: A dangerous health policy fad that won't die. *STAT*, January 30, 2018.

CHAPTER 8

INADEQUATE OVERSIGHT OF HEALTH CARE ACROSS THE MEDICAL-INDUSTRIAL COMPLEX

After all we've seen in previous chapters about how poor access is to affordable health care of good quality for much of the U. S. population, wouldn't you think that government should play a more active role in better regulating our so-called system's downsides? Think again, as we will soon see.

This chapter has three goals: (1) to look across many parts of our health care system to assess the extent of regulation in each area; (2) to briefly discuss increasing deregulation under the Trump administration, with the FDA a poster child of inadequate oversight; and (3) to summarize four adverse impacts of reduced accountability of U. S. health care while rewarding corporate interests.

"Regulation" of U. S. Health Care
Private Insurers

We have many examples of profit-driven feeding at the public trough often bordering on and becoming fraud. Here are some of them.

- Despite hopes by Congress in the early 2000s that private Medicare Advantage could be more efficient and provide better coverage than traditional Medicare, that wishful

thinking has long been exposed as a lie. Medicare
Advantage insurers, including the giant UnitedHealth
Group, have been bilking the program for many years
by gaming the payment system, typically by overstating
the risk scores of payments in order to gain higher
reimbursement. [1,2]

- Private Medicaid plans are equally unable to prove
  themselves more efficient than their public counterparts.
  Overpayments to privatized Medicaid plans are endemic
  in more than 30 states, often involving unnecessary or
  duplicative payments to providers. [3,4]
- Private Medicaid plans typically deny necessary care
  through sub-contractors (often owned by equity firms) in
  order to gain higher revenues for themselves and shareholders. Patients also have longer waits for care in inadequate physician networks. [5,6]

Hospitals

The federal government handed off most of the accreditation
function to meet safety conditions in hospitals to an Illinois-based
Joint Commission back in 1965 when Medicare and Medicaid
were enacted. Most hospitals pay the Commission for periodic
inspections to retain their accreditation in order to continue to receive reimbursement for their services. As the largest of private
accreditors, the Joint Commission has some conflicts of interest,
with 20 of its 32 members executives at health systems it accredits
or work at parent corporations of such systems. Not surprisingly,
almost all inspected hospitals retain accreditation despite identifi-
cation of serious ongoing safety violations. [7]

An investigation by the *Wall Street Journal* found that less than one percent of more than 100 psychiatric hospitals overseen by the Joint Commission in fiscal years 2014 and 2015 were denied full accreditation even when safety violations were found that included preventable deaths, abuse, or sexual assault of patients.[8]

Nursing homes

There are some 15,000 nursing homes in the country, two thirds of which are private, where profits rule the realm. Nursing homes receive about $500 a day for a patient on traditional Medicare, compared to $430 a day for a Medicare patient in a managed care plan and just $200 a day for a Medicaid patient. When sicker patients require more care and when reimbursement becomes limited, nursing homes frequently discharge and evict patients as they game a weakly regulated system for higher profits. These examples are typical of a growing national problem. [9]

- *Deborah Zwaschka-Blansfield, 59, was told that her insurance would no longer pay six weeks after the lower half of her left leg was amputated. The nursing home, north of Sacramento, wanted to release her to a homeless shelter or pay for a week in a motel, despite her inability to walk and being at high risk for a fall.*

- *Alan Schoen, 58, after two hospitalizations after a fall and later with a bladder infection and pancreatitis, was told that his insurance would soon stop paying and that he should move to an assisted living facility, where he would receive less needed care. As he said at the time, "They are running a business. I get that, but it seems they forget the patient element in all of this."*

- *Gloria Single, 82, became more agitated with Alzheimer's, and was discharged from a California nursing home where she lived with her husband. Although she won an appeal, the nursing home still would not accept her back. As her attorney said, "They don't take you back and there are no consequences."*

In recent years, private equity firms have moved into the business of "serving" some of the nation's poorest and most vulnerable people. These firms profit by pooling money from investors, borrowing even more, and then buying, revamping, and selling off nursing home companies. The Carlyle Group, one of the richest private-equity firms in the world, did just that in buying and then neglecting ManorCare, the second largest nursing home chain in the country. Soon after buying the company, hundreds of layoffs were announced and staffing was inadequate, leading to increasing numbers of serious health-code violations and harm to patients. The company finally had to file for bankruptcy, but only after investors had extracted $1.3 billion from it. [10]

The Trump administration is missing in action on regulating nursing homes. While claiming its intent to address improper evictions as part of its push toward deregulation, it has scaled back the use of fines against nursing homes that harm patients. [11] Moreover, in February 2018, the administration imposed an 18-month moratorium on imposing fines or denials of federal payments when nursing homes fail to meet such requirements as ensuring that they have adequate staffing or are using psychotropic drugs correctly. [12]

Assisted Living

A 2018 report by the Government Accountability Office (GAO) found that more than 330,000 Medicaid beneficiaries are receiving care in a growing lucrative assisted living industry with almost no standards and little oversight by federal or state authorities. Only 22 states were able to furnish information on "critical incidents—cases of potential or actual harm." In one year, those states reported a total of 22,900 such incidents, including physical, emotional, or sexual abuse of residents. To this date, the Centers for Medicare and Medicaid Services (CMS) has provided little guidance to deal with this situation. [13]

Surgery Centers

There are more than 5,600 surgery centers in the country, an industry catering to outpatient surgery with the false idea that they can save some of the costs of inpatient hospital care. Medicare noted in 2007 that these centers "have neither patient safety standards consistent with those in place for hospitals, nor are they required to have the trained staff and equipment needed to provide the breadth or intensity of care . . ." There are conflicts of interest that further endanger patients since federal law still allows surgery center doctors to steer patients to facilities they own, instead of to a full-service hospital. This can increase patients' risks and allow physicians to "triple-dip"—increase their income by performing the surgery as well as receiving further income through facility fees as an owner and investor in the facility. [14]

Surgery centers are still woefully under regulated despite an ongoing trend of their taking on patients of higher risk and their poor track record over many years. When emergencies arise, surgery centers call 911 and send these patients to nearby hospitals, as occurred for at least 7,000 patients in the year that ended in September 2017. A recent investigation by *Kaiser Health News* reporters and *USA TODAY Network* found that 260 patients have died since 2013 after inadequate care following in-and-out procedures in surgery centers across the country. Here is just one of these tragic patient stories. [15]

> *Paulina Tam, 58, the mother of three who had completed careers as a nurse and educator, planned to travel with her husband of 32 years after having surgery in a surgery center for two discs in the upper spine. Four hours after the procedure, with the surgeon and anesthesiologist already gone for the day, she had difficulty breathing. No staff could intubate her or otherwise establish an airway. After a 24-minute transfer to the nearest hospital, she arrived without a pulse, was put on life support, and died the next morning.*

Despite this unacceptable lack of accountability over the years, state and federal oversight of surgery centers is still grossly inadequate. Even in the unusual circumstance where Medicare issues its most severe penalty—involuntary decertification—state accreditation agencies can still allow their continued operation, even awarding gold seals for "quality" of care. [16]

Dialysis clinics

Devita, one of the largest for-profit chains of dialysis clinics in the country, operates more than 2,500 clinics, including 292 clinics in California, one-half of all such clinics in the state. The chain, now owned by UnitedHealth Group, with $1.5 to $1.6 billion a year in profits, has been under fire for years over its high charges and poor patient outcomes. Proposition 8, a ballot measure in November 2018 in California intended to regulate Devita, failed as the industry poured in some $111 million in its defense. Also in 2018, a federal jury in Colorado awarded $383 million in 2018 to the families of three of its dialysis patients in wrongful death lawsuits. [17]

For-profit dialysis clinics have increased their profits for many years by using shorter dialysis periods and reusing manufactured dialyzers that are labeled for single use in just one patient. [18] Compared to their not-for-profit counterparts, they have had death rates 30 percent higher, with 20 percent less use of transplants. [19]

Drug industry

Big PhRMA continues its long track record as the poster child for irresponsible and exploitive practices that place profits for their CEOs and shareholders above the public interest. Drug companies continue to raise their prices to what the traffic can bear, even as they lobby hard against any regulation. These examples make the point:

- The price of Mylan's EpiPen, a lifesaving treatment for emergency allergic reactions, increased by more than sixfold over several years without any improvement in the treatment. [20]
- The price of Duraprim, often used by patients with HIV, increased by 5,500 percent from $13.50 to $750 per tablet in 2015. Martin Shkreli, the CEO of the manufacturer, was later found guilty on two counts of security fraud. [21]

- Nirmal Mulye, founder and president of Nostrum Pharmaceuticals, after raising the price of the antibiotic Nitrofurantoin, used for urinary tract infections, by more than 400 percent, claimed that this increase is his "moral requirement to make money when you can." [22]

- The drug industry has long touted the safety of hydrocodone and oxycodone for chronic pain. Today, the opioid epidemic has claimed the lives of more than 200,000 Americans, more than three times the number of U. S. military deaths in the Vietnam War. Federal lawsuits have been brought in five states alleging fraud, racketeering and unjust profits by defendant companies.[23]

- A recent study looked at county-specific data across the country, finding that the more marketing dollars were spent by drug companies to influence doctors in a county, the higher the rates of their prescribing opioids and the more overdose deaths occurred in that county. [24]

- A recent report found that criminal penalties against pharmaceutical companies have all but disappeared since 1991 for such illegal conduct as drug pricing fraud, kickback payments to hospitals and other providers, and concealing results of company-sponsored studies. [25]

- Secret deals involving drug makers and pharmacy benefit managers, such as CVS Caremark and Express Scripts, drive higher prices for prescription drugs without any public awareness as they accelerate through corporate mergers. [26] A recent report in Kentucky found that PBMs there, through a process known as "spread pricing," charge pharmacies fees that are then billed back to the State Medicaid program, including hidden profits of $123.5 million retained in 2018. [27]

- The December 2017 $1.5 trillion tax bill passed by the Republican-led Congress and signed by Trump was a huge windfall for the drug industry through cuts in the corporate tax rate from 35 percent to 21 percent and other provisions. The question at first was whether consumers would see lower costs of their drug products. No way! Drug prices kept going up as drug makers spent much of the windfall on buying back stocks and issuing dividends to the benefit of shareholders, not patients. [28]

As the above examples reveal, wherever we look across the medical-industrial complex, the story is the same—profiteering on the backs of sick people, their families, and taxpayers. Such regulations as we have are completely inadequate. While this has been a problem for many years, it is much worse now under Trump's policy of deregulation across the government.

Deregulation of Health Care under the Trump Administration

Deregulation of health care over Trump's first two years in office fits the pattern of what's happening across the board in other sectors, including safety, labor, financial, and environmental sectors. All this is based on a false claim that deregulation will somehow get us on a better track in this country. He issued an executive order just ten days after his inauguration calling for government agencies to kill two rules for every one they propose.

Trump's Cabinet was carefully selected to pursue a goal of "deconstruction of the administrative state," a policy strongly supported by the Freedom Caucus, many trade organizations, and corporate lobbyists. [29] Another executive order was issued titled

"Ethical Commitments by Executive Branch Appointees," but it was just window dressing that lowered ethical standards. Six months later, there were 74 lobbyists working in his administration, 49 of whom in agencies they once lobbied on behalf of clients. [30] Without regard for that executive order, Trump has issued many waivers of these ethical standards, usually to individuals who had been retained by for-profit clients and dealt with matters which could benefit those former clients. [31]

The Food and Drug Administration (FDA) has for many years been a classic example of inadequate regulation of pharmaceutical companies. Drug makers are always seeking quick approval of their products. However, almost one-third of drugs approved by the FDA from 2000 to 2010 were withdrawn from the market due to safety concerns and risk to the public. [32]

With support of the industry, the Prescription Drug User Fee Act (PDUFA) was enacted in 1992 whereby drug companies pay the bulk of the FDA's budget in order to speed up the regulatory process. That obviously creates a potential fox-in-the-hen-house conflict of interest. Since 1992, Big PhRMA has contributed $7.67 billion to the FDA in user fees, with the amounts accelerating in recent years. [33] (Figure 8.1)

Remarkably, the FDA does not require evidence of added efficacy or safety over comparison drugs. About 90 percent of newly approved drugs bring few or no clinical benefits, while most drug research is aimed to generate new patents of minor variations in order to charge patent protected prices. [34] The FDA is increasingly using industry-friendly expedited development and approval pathways with greater emphasis on post-marketing drug data supplied by the companies. A recent article by physicians calls these approval standards too low and post-approval evaluation too lax.[35]

FIGURE 8.1

BIG PhRMA CONTRIBUTIONS TO FDA IN USER FEES

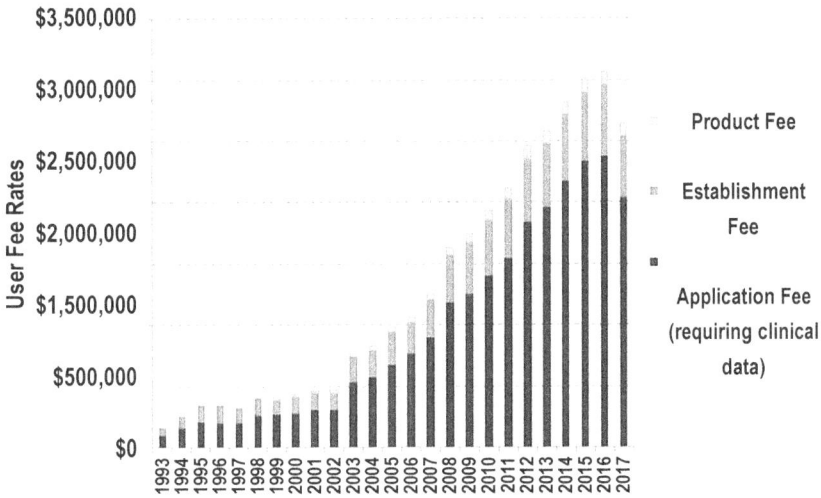

Sources: Avalere Analysis of Prescription Drug User Fee Rates. 1993 - 2017

This current major problem shows how little confidence we can have in the regulatory process. As the opioid crisis continues largely unchecked across the country, a large highly lucrative industry has emerged testing urine for drugs. Fraud has become a big problem as many doctor-owned testing clinics charge high billings to Medicare and other payers. Comprehensive Pain Specialists, as one example, has a network of 54 such clinics that billed Medicare at least $11 million for urine and related tests in 2014; one nurse practitioner in a Tennessee clinic single-handedly generated $1.1 million in Medicare billings that year. Today, there are still no national standards for who gets tested, for what drugs, and how often.[36]

This patient's story illustrates this ongoing unaddressed problem.

> *Elizabeth Moreno, 30, had back surgery in late 2015.*
> *After the surgery, her surgeon prescribed an opioid for pain*
> *and what seemed like a follow-up urine drug test. She and*
> *her physician father were shocked soon thereafter when they*
> *received a bill for $17,850 from a laboratory for the urine*
> *test, which checked for many drugs, including PCP, an ille-*
> *gal hallucinogenic drug. Experts doubted the need for the*
> *test, which was considered fraudulent. A reporter for Kaiser*
> *Health News noted that the urine testing boom consumes*
> *billions of dollars every year, often for needless tests at ex-*
> *orbitant prices.* [37]

Adverse Impacts of Deregulation on Health Care

Here are four major adverse impacts of industry-friendly deregulation, all predictable in our deregulated profit-driven marketplace.

1. Higher costs resulting in less access to affordable care

In this deregulated environment, the profit-driven medical industrial complex makes it impossible to contain the accelerating costs of U. S. health care.

The health care industry spends at least $30 *billion* a year marketing its wares, which drives more testing and more treatments. [38] The electronics industry is mining health care for new profits, ranging from the Welt smart belt (which monitors the time one spends sitting and the number of steps taken) to RxPense, (a high-tech pill dispenser with bells, whistles, and even a recording camera!). [39]

2. Increase in inappropriate and unnecessary care, often harming patients.

It is estimated that about one-third of all health services provided each year in this country are inappropriate or unnecessary. We live in a culture of over-treatment which is often harmful to patients. A recent study published in the highly respected journal *Lancet,* as one example, reports that cardiac stents placed so commonly for stable chest pain don't provide more relief of symptoms than drug therapy and that one in fifty patients experience serious complications, such as a heart attack, bleeding, or even death. [40]

3. Weakened scientific basis for health care services

An important 2017 book from the Princeton University Press, *Unhealthy Politics: The Battle over Evidence-Based Medicine*, documents how many common treatments are not based on sound science, and go into widespread use before being rigorously evaluated. It also shows how frequently patients are harmed as a result and how inadequate the response by our government has been. [41]

4. Increased corporate crime and misconduct

As part of its broad attack on regulation, the Trump administration has reduced penalties for corporate crime and misconduct of the nation's 100 most profitable corporations from about $17 billion a year during the Obama administration to just $1.1 billion in Trump's first year in office. [42]

As these adverse impacts continue without effective oversight, CEOs, shareholders and investors thrive at the expense of patients, families and taxpayers, and as S & P 500 health stocks lead the pack.

Conclusion

Accountability is inadequate all across the board in the Trump administration, worse now than ever before. Trump's deregulatory policies fuel profiteering by corporate stakeholders and higher costs, resulting in less access to affordable care and lower quality of care as corporate interests pursue profits over service. Excesses of for-profit health care become more obvious all the time.

There is an urgent need for greater accountability and a larger role of government in regulating health care, as we will deal with in Part III. For now, however, it's time to move to the next two chapters in Part II to see what is left of a safety net for health care.

References:

1. Walsh, MW. A whistle-blower tells of health insurers bilking Medicare. *New York Times*, May 15, 2017.
2. Schulte, F. Audits of some Medicare Advantage plans reveal pervasive overcharging. *NPR Now* KPLU, August 29, 2016: 1.
3. Herman, B. Medicaid's unmanaged managed care. *Modern Healthcare*, April 30, 2016.
4. Bailey, M. Seniors suffer amid widespread fraud by Medicaid caretakers. *Kaiser Health News*, November 7, 2016.
5. Terhune, C. Coverage denied: Medicaid patients suffer as layers of private companies profit. *Kaiser Health News*, January 3, 2019.
6. Himmelstein, DU, Woolhandler, S. The post-launch problem: The Affordable Act's persistently high administrative costs. *Health Affairs Blog*, May 27, 2017.
7. Armour, S. Hospitals keep 'gold seal' despite woes. *Wall Street Journal*, September 9-10, 2017.
8. Armour, S. Troubled hospitals maintain credentials. *Wall Street Journal*, December 27, 2018.
9. Bernard, TS, Pear, R. Complaints about nursing home evictions rise, and regulators take note. *New York Times*, February 22, 2018.

10. Whoriskey, P, Keating, D. Overdoses, bedsores, broken bones: What happened when a private-equity firm sought to care for society's most vulnerable? *The Washington Post*, November 25, 2018.

11. Weixel, N. Dems seek reversal of nursing home regulatory rollback. *The Hill*, February 20, 2018.

12. Gorman, A. Weak oversight blamed for poor care at California nursing homes going unchecked. *Kaiser Health News*, May 4, 2018.

13. Pear, R. U. S. pays billions for 'assisted living', but what does it get? *New York Times*, February 3, 2018.

14. Jewett, C, Alesia, M. As surgery centers boom, patients are paying with their lives. *Kaiser Health News*, March 2, 2018.

15. Ibid # 14.

16. Jewett, C. Despite red flags at surgery centers, overseers award gold seals. *Kaiser Health News*, September 20, 2018.

17. Young, S. Dialysis giant Devita defends itself in court and at the polls. *Kaiser Health News*, October 29, 2018.

18. Himmelstein, DU, Woolhandler, S, Hellander, I. *Bleeding the Patient: The Consequences of Corporate Health Care.* Monroe, ME. *Common Courage Press, 2001.*

19. Geyman, JP. *The Corporate Transformation of Health Care: Can the Public Interest Still Be Served?* New York. *Springer Publishing Company*, 2004, p. 228.

20. Court, E. Mylan's epi-pen price increases are Valeant-like in size, Shkreli-like in approach. *Marketwatch*, August 18, 2016.

21. Emett, A. A Big PhRMA raises price of cancer drug by 1,400 percent. *Nation of Change*, December 27, 2017.

22. PhRMA exec claims 'moral requirement' to raise drug price 400%. Dispatches. *The Progressive Populist*, October 15, 2018, p. 22.

23. Randazzo, S. New front in opioid lawsuits: Rise in insurance premiums. *Wall Street Journal,* May 3, 2018.

24. Knight, V. County by county, researchers link opioid deaths to drugmakers' marketing. *Kaiser Health News*, January 18, 2019.

25. Prupis, N. Penalties for PhRMA crimes have all but disappeared, report finds. *Public Citizen News*, May/June 2018, p. 11.

26. Serafini, M, Barrett, R. Secret deals drive higher prescription drug costs. *Tarbell*, May 24, 2018.

27. The Office of U. S. Senator Cory A. Booker. With New Tax Savings, Drug Companies Start by Rewarding Shareholders, Not Patients Struggling with Skyrocketing Prices, April 9, 2018.

28. Silverman, E. Kentucky finds PBMs are benefiting from a lucrative profit center. *STAT*, February 21, 2019.

29. Steinzor, R. The war on regulation. *The American Prospect*, Spring 2017, pp. 72-76.

30. Nazaryan, A. The swamp runneth over. *Newsweek*, November 10, 2017.

31. Lipton, E, Ivory, D. Lobbyists, industry lawyers were granted ethics waivers to work in Trump administration. *New York Times*, June 8, 2017.

32. Lupkin, S. Nearly 1 in 3 recent FDA drug approvals followed by major safety actions. *Kaiser Health News*, May 9, 2017.

33. Ramsey, L, Friedman, L. The government agency in charge of approving drugs gets a surprising amount of money from the companies that make them. *Business Insider*, August 17, 2016.

34. Light, DW, Caplan, AL. Trump blames free riding states for high U. S. drug prices. *British Medical Journal*, March 16, 2018.

35. Kesselheim, AS, Woloshin, S, Lu, Z. Physicians' perspectives on FDA approval standards and off label drug marketing. *JAMA Internal Medicine*, January 22, 2019.

36. Schulte, F, Lucas, E. Liquid gold: Pain doctors soak up profits by screening urine for drugs. *Kaiser Health News,* November 6, 2017.

37. Schulte, F. Pain hits after surgery when a doctor's daughter is stunned by $17,850 urine test. *Kaiser Health News*, February 16, 2018.

38. Szabo, L. Health care industry spends $30B a year pushing its wares, from drugs to stem cell treatment. *Kaiser Health News*, January 8, 2019.

39. Taub, E. The electronics industry sees money in your health. *Kaiser Health News*, January 16, 2019.

40. Belluz, J. Thousands of heart patients get stents that may do more harm than good. *Vox*, November 6, 2017.

41. Gerber, AS, Patashnik, EM, Dowling, CM. *Unhealthy Politics: The Battle over Evidence-Based Medicine, Princeton University Press*, 2017.

42. Johnson, J. Tracking tool shows fines for corporate misconduct have plummeted under Trump. *Common Dreams*, February 13, 2018.

PART II

THE LONG GONE SAFETY NET

What we deal with in our work, quite apart from the extremes of genocide, is a variant of that: "Lives less worthy of life." When we say that the poor have a mortality rate that is multiple times the rate of the rich, when we say that poor children die in our country and in the developing world at rates far higher than those of the better off, we are saying that we permit a condition which in effect says that they are less worthy of life. We are sending this message because we let it happen, because we have social politics that almost assure that it will happen, and we let it happen stubbornly and continually.

—H. Jack Geiger, M.D., Founding member and past president of Physicians for Human Rights, past president of Physicians for Social Responsibility, and pioneering developer of community health centers.

Source: Why we do what we do, speech. *Doctors for Global Health,* August, 2002

CHAPTER 9

MYTHS, MEMES, LIES AND POLITICS

We're going to have insurance for everybody. People can expect to have great health care. It will be in a much simplified form. Must less expensive and much better.

—President Donald Trump before his inauguration,
The Washington Post, January 15, 2017

The above lie is one of the more than 10,000 lies told by Trump over the first twenty-seven months of his administration, as recorded by *The Washington Post.* These lies and disinformation by him and his administration, together with long-term myths and memes perpetuated by conservatives about U. S. health care over many years, continue to confuse the public and distort the political debate over how to reform our health care system for the common good.

This chapter has two goals: (1) to sort through some of the major myths, memes, and lies that continue to distort the debate over health care reform; and (2) to describe how these have been translated into health care policies of the Trump administration.

Some Myths, Memes and Lies
1. Everyone gets care anyway.

This is a common myth, now a meme, among many people who assume that people can always get health care, even if uninsured or underinsured. Isn't that what emergency rooms and urgent care centers are for? The bald fact, however, is that many millions of Americans cannot afford to gain access to such facilities, and even if they do, their care will be inadequate in terms of comprehensiveness or continuity. Emergency rooms deal only with the single main presenting complaint, and have difficulty arranging follow-up for acute conditions in a system without enough primary care physicians and all too many physicians not accepting new patients unless they are well insured.

2. We don't ration care in this country.

This is a common notion that disregards the everyday experience of many patients who cannot gain access to necessary care in our market-based system that denies care, not just to the 28 million uninsured but also to tens of millions more who have some kind of insurance but are underinsured. Ironically, purveyors of this myth often discredit other advanced nations with *universal* health care, by claiming that *they* ration care!

Yes, we ration care based on ability to pay, not by medical necessity. Beyond unaffordability of care, these are some of the other ways that we ration care in this country:

- Denial of services by insurers.
- Disenrollment of sicker patients in privatized Medicare and Medicaid programs.
- Restrictive coverage by insurers for women's health care and mental health.
- Insurers placing cancer and other specialized drugs in top tiers that are unaffordable even for the insured.

3. Consumer directed health care, whereby patients have more 'skin in the game,' will save money.

There has been a long-standing assumption, even by many health economists, that people will overuse health care services because they have insurance. This belief is based on the theory of *moral hazard*, which has been used by supporters of consumer-driven health care (CDHC), the prevailing policy that assumes that patients will make more prudent choices if they have more "skin in the game" through larger co-payments, deductibles, and other restrictions. More than two decades of experience with CDHC in this country, however, have resulted in too much of our population forgoing essential care and having worse outcomes. In a 2007 paper published in the *International Journal of Health Services*, I laid out these other reasons to put this myth to rest, all even more relevant today:

- *Health care is a basic human need, not just another commodity for sale on the open market.*
- *Instead of enhancing choice, CDHC usually reduces individuals' choice of health care.*
- *Moral hazard-based assumptions underlying CDHC have always failed to rein in surging costs of health care.*
- *High-deductible CDHC plans with increased cost-sharing segment the market by favoring the healthy and avoiding the sick.*
- *The more that CDHC succeeds in attracting healthier people to its plans, the greater the need for public safety net coverage, already increasingly frayed by budget deficits.* [1]

4. The private sector is more efficient and can fix system problems better than the public sector.

Unfortunately, many economists still think that health care markets work like other markets, where competition can rein in prices and patients can shop for the best deal, such as they would in buying a car. We have learned over the last 40 years, however, that this is not true. Patients usually don't really know their needs, urgency of time is often a controlling factor, information is not available about costs of care, and consolidation of corporate providers tends to increase costs and financial barriers to care while restricting patients' choices. We end up with more bureaucracy and higher administrative costs in our mostly for-profit multi-payer private insurer financing system than any other advanced country in the world.

As just one example of how poorly the private system is in dealing with an important challenge to develop electronic health records (EHRs) that are better, safer and cheaper, consider our experience over the last ten years. Business incentives to make more money have resulted in chaos among competing EHR systems that do not talk to each other, are so complex and time consuming for physicians that they contribute to physician burnout, and are resistant to interoperability. Patients have to struggle to get their own records, with little more than one-half of hospitals offering patients an option to receive their entire medical record. Many health care providers are reluctant to freely exchange such information due to concerns of losing patients to competing physicians or hospitals, which created the term "leakage" for lost revenue. [2]

Perhaps as a "solution" that raises another problem, new concerns about patients' privacy are now being raised by new efforts by giant corporations such as the insurer Cigna and EHR companies Epic Systems and Cerner Corp., intended to consolidate information like diagnoses and laboratory diagnoses for patients to access through their computers or smart-phones. Such consolidated information is not subject to the Health Information Privacy and Accountability Act of 1996 (HIPAA) [3]

5. States can resolve health care system problems better than the federal government.

As we know, a high priority for the GOP and Trump after the 2016 elections was to shift responsibility for much of our health care from the federal government to the states. After the failure of GOP legislation to repeal the ACA, they granted more waivers to the states to get around the ACA's constraints. The philosophy held that the states, being closer to the needs of their populations, could do the job better. State block grants for Medicaid and other safety net programs were proposed as a way to bring down the federal deficit (which grew by $1.5 trillion by the December 2017 "tax cut" bill!), and decrease federal funds for these programs by expecting states to shoulder more of their costs. One study found that the federal government would save $150 billion by 2022 if Medicaid were funded by per capita block grants. [4]

Were this approach to become widespread, the results are predictable—state Medicaid programs would be gutted, ending a more than 50-year social contract with poor and lower-income Americans. States would opt out of some or most of the 10 essential benefits required of insurers by the ACA (including letting insurers deny coverage based on pre-existing conditions). As already stressed state budgets fall short of their program needs, private contractors will entice them with promises that they can work cheaper, better, and faster. And we all know what that means— higher costs as they profiteer new taxpayer funded markets with little or no accountability. [5]

6. *"We have the best economy in 50 years."*

Trump has boasted on multiple occasions that his administration has brought us the best economy in 50 years. That, of course, is another blatant lie as inequality in our society has reached new levels. Robert Reich, professor of public policy at the University of California Berkeley and author of a recent book, *The Common Good*, makes these points about our current circumstances:

- Over 80 percent of the stock market is owned by the richest 10 percent of Americans, so most people haven't partaken of the recent stock market boom.
- Despite the conservative theory of "trickle down" economics, hourly wages adjusted for inflation are not much higher now than they were 40 years ago.
- Trump and the GOP still refuse to raise the federal minimum wage, which is stuck at $7.25 an hour.
- While unemployment is down to 3.7 percent, jobs are less secure than ever, with contract workers doing one out of every five jobs in America and not receiving usual employers' benefits.
- With skyrocketing housing costs, many Americans are paying a third or more of their paychecks in rent or mortgages.

Reich further observes:

> *Too often, discussions about "the economy" focus on overall statistics about growth, the stock market and unemployment. But most Americans don't live in that economy. They live in a personal economy that has more to do with wages, job security, commutes to and from work, and the costs of housing, health care, drugs, education and home insurance. . . . Instead of an "economic boom," most Americans are experiencing declines in these dimension of their lives.* [6]

7. Medicare for All is a socialistic plan by the government to take over health care.

As single-payer Medicare for All took center stage before and after the 2018 election campaigns, attack dogs from the GOP and Trump administration were released to dispense their lies. Disingenuous and false claims from the right include assertions that this would be a socialist government takeover of health care, that it would break the bank, that Medicare would be destroyed, that people would lose benefits and choice of their doctors, and that wait times would go way up. [7]

Trump declared that Medicare for All would eviscerate Medicare, rob seniors of benefits they have paid for their entire lives, and end up being Medicare for none. He vowed that he would protect Medicare from the Democrats! [8] Seema Verma, CMS director of Medicare in the Trump administration, chimed in: "We only have to look at some of Medicare's major problems to know that it's a bad idea." [9] On another occasion, she came up with this further "wisdom:" "Putting more people in the program is not going to solve the problem, and actually threatens the focus and security of the program for seniors." [10]

These, of course, are all bald-faced lies intended to distort the real debate we need to have over health care reform. The facts are clear—universal coverage through Medicare for All will bring comprehensive health benefits to all U.S. residents, with full choice of providers, who remain in private practice. That is hardly socialism. It will be much more efficient than today's health care maelstrom, and more affordable for patients, families, and taxpayers than the current exploitive market-based non-system.

We can achieve universal coverage through big savings from eliminating the private insurance middlemen that now drain many billions of dollars annually from our health care system for marketing, accounting, executives' bonuses and profits—all of no value to actual health care. In 2018, private health insurers' overhead totaled more than $256 billion, 12 percent of their premium revenue and five times the administrative overhead of traditional Medicare. [11]

All U. S. residents would pay into the new system through a progressive tax base, whereby 95 percent would pay less than they do now for health insurance and care. According to a recent study, lower and middle income families will pay much less for health care with Medicare for All, while the top 5 percent of families with annual incomes more than $400,000 will pay only 5.6 percent more. (Table 9.1) [12]

TABLE 9.1
Health Care Spending by Family Income
Under Medicare for All

	Health care spending as share of income		3. Change in health care spending as share of income
	1. Existing system	2. Medicare for All	(= column 2 – column 1)
Low-income families			
$13,000 in income with Medicaid	3.5%	-0.1%	-3.7%
$35,000 in income, uninsured	2.5%	1.7%	-0.8%
Middle-income families: $60,000 in income			
Underinsured	8.0%	1.6%	-6.4%
Individually insured	15.5%	1.6%	-14.0%
Insured by employer	4.2%	1.6%	-2.6%
High-income families			
Top 20 percent: $221,000 in income	-0.1%	3.7%	+3.9%
Top 5 percent: $401,000 in income	-0.9%	4.7%	+5.6%

Source: Pollin, R, Heintz, J, Arno, P et al. *In-Depth Analysis by Team of UMass Amherst Economists Shows Viability of Medicare for All*. Amherst, MA, November 30, 2018.

Politics of Health Care under Trump

Here are some of the major approaches that the Trump administration has taken, based on myths, memes, and lies, to address the ongoing barriers to access and affordability of health care in this country.

1. "Stabilize the health insurance market."

Trump's October 2017 Executive Order ordered governmental agencies, including the DHHS, Labor, and Treasury, to loosen restrictions on selling low-cost, short-term health insurance and association health plans; encourage tax-free employer contributions through health-reimbursement accounts (HRAs); and propose other ways to increase choice and reduce consolidation in the health care market. Other big changes early in his administration were the repeal of the individual mandate as part of the 2017 GOP tax cut bill and stopping CSR subsidies, which created more uncertainty in health insurance markets.

Instead of stabilizing markets, they remain more volatile than ever as insurers explore new ways of profiting from marketing "insurance" with less actuarial value and less reliability.

2. Give more flexibility to the states.

A 365-page rule issued in October 2017 by Seema Verma, as CMS head, allowed states to determine how essential benefits should be defined, let insurers spend more of their premium dollars on administration and profits, and relaxed the threshold for state regulators to review premium increases from 10 to 15 percent. [13] Later moves by CMS extended state waivers allowing them to establish work requirements for Medicaid beneficiaries, set caps on number of years of Medicaid coverage, use drug screening to determine eligibility, and set premiums that are unaffordable for low-income people. [14]

In calling for "an unprecedented level of flexibility" for states to design their own Medicaid programs, Verma's intent is to slash Medicaid rolls and reduce federal funding for Medicaid. Before joining the Trump administration, she changed Indiana's Medicaid program by requiring enrollees to make income-based contributions to a health savings account, akin to premiums, or lose benefits and coverage. [15] By early 2018, almost three-quarters of states were involved in Medicaid demonstration programs, such as subcontracting to private managed care firms and requiring enrollees to pay monthly premiums. But the General Accounting Office has found, not surprisingly, that evaluations of these programs by states and CMS are very weak. [16] More flexability to states is resulting in less health care for their residents.

3. Further privatization of Medicare and Medicaid

The Trump administration has aggressively promoted further privatization of Medicare Advantage from the start, despite our long experience that private plans are more expensive, less efficient, more restrictive of choice of physician and hospital, and have administrative costs about five times higher than traditional Medicare. [17] Private Medicare plans have gamed the system for high overpayments of taxpayer dollars from the government over many years as corporate stakeholders lobby Congress for their continuation. [18] A 2017 article by Sam Baker in *Axios Vitals* described the startup of a new private Medicare insurer, Devoted Health, observing that:

> *Medicare Advantage is where the big money is. The ACA marketplaces grab a lot of headlines, but they are a blip on the radar when compared with the hundreds of billions of dollars tied up in private Medicare plans and care for seniors.* [19]

Private Medicaid plans follow the same pattern as private Medicare plans. Compared to their public counterparts, privatized Medicaid programs have longer waits for care, inadequate physician networks, and denials of many treatments, even as insurers take in higher profits. [20] They also have worse outcomes of care than their public counterparts. [21] Almost three-quarters of the 73 million Americans on Medicaid are now in private managed care plans, whereby states pay subcontractors monthly fixed amounts for each enrollee. The more these plans can skimp on care and deny services, the more money they make. The State of California has found that one Long Beach company delayed or denied care for at least 1,400 enrollees. Medicaid officials have no authority over these subcontractors. [22]

4. Short-term health insurance plans

A final rule released by the Trump administration in August 2018 relaxed all of the ACA's requirements for insurers, allowing them to market short-term less expensive plans up to one year that cover very little. These short-term plans typically exclude coverage for preventive care, maternity care, pediatric care, rehabilitative services and mental health services. They set annual and lifetime limits, and can be renewed for up to two more years unless enrollees develop a new deniable health condition. They attract younger, healthier people with low premiums, but are best considered "junk insurance." [23] Predictably, however, insurers make big profits on these short-term plans, paying out only about two-thirds of premium revenues on medical care, while brokers pocket commissions of 20 percent. [24]

5. Expansion of association health plans

Association health plans (AHPs) have been touted by Trump as another way to get around the ACA by allowing small employers to band together in associations as a means to gain health coverage for their employees at lower cost. AHPs do not comply with the ACA's requirements for coverage, expose enrollees to high out-of-pocket costs, and siphon off healthier individuals, thereby further segmenting the risk pool. [25] The National Federation of Independent Business (NFIB) has promoted this idea for two decades, but has recently given them up as impractical, too complex, and not worth the effort. [26]

6. Expand health savings accounts (HSAs)

Republicans have long touted HSAs as a good way for Americans to put aside money, tax-free, to pay for unexpected future expenses. The problem for most people, however, is that they don't have enough money in savings to use these accounts. Almost one-half of Americans cannot cover a $400 emergency expense. [27] Only upper income people can benefit from HSAs.

Instead of being useful for most people, HSAs have become a large and very profitable industry on Wall Street. In the six months after the November 2016 elections, the shares of HSA provider HealthEquity increased by about 35 percent, becoming one of the best performing stocks. Optum Bank, the industry leader, is owned by UnitedHealth Group, the nation's largest health insurer, and manages some $7 billion for its 3 million accounts. [28]

Although the above policies were promoted to the public as improving their health care, they were all misguided based on long experience. Richard Eskow, senior fellow at Campaign for America's Future, sees through the lies by the GOP and Trump administration in this way:

> *Give them less and make them think it's more. That's the Republican Party's goal with "TrumpCare." Why? They're doing it to provide enormous tax breaks to the wealthiest among us, after we have already achieved levels of inequality not seen since the Roaring Twenties or the Gilded Age of the Nineteenth Century.* [29]

Conclusion

So much for the lies and actions of the GOP and Trump administration about health care. In the next chapter we will see how misguided and harmful they are to a deteriorating safety net for so much of our population.

References

1.   Geyman, JP. Moral hazard and consumer-driven health care: A fundamentally flawed concept. *Intl J Health Services* 37 (2), 2007.
2.   Schulte, F, Fry, E. Death by a 1,000 clicks: Where electronic health records went wrong. *Kaiser Health News*, March 18, 2019.
3.   Mathews, AW. Rush into health apps spurs privacy fears. *Wall Street Journal*, April 3, 2019: B 1.
4.   Hellman, J. Study: Medicaid block grants would save feds $150 billion. *The Hill*, February 6, 2017.
5.   Cohen, D. TrumpCare will be a gold rush for private contractors. *In the Public Interest*, March 16, 2017.
6.   Reich, R. The truth about the Trump economy. *The Progressive Populist*, November 15, 2018, p. 13.
7.   Alonzo-Zaldivar. AP FACT CHECK: Trump distorts Democrats' health care ideas. *AP News*, October 9, 2018.
8.   Trump, DJ., as quoted by Waldman, P. Trump's *USA Today* piece reveals the GOP's massive problem on health care. *The Washington Post*, December 28, 2018.
9.   Galewitz, P. Medicare for All? CMS chief warns program has enough problems already. *Kaiser Health News*, October 16, 2018.
10. Minemyer, P. Verma, Azar take aim at "Medicare for All" proposals. *Fierce Healthcare*, October 5, 2018.proposals.
11. Woolhandler, S, Himmelstein, DU. What Trump gets wrong about Medicare for All. *CNN*, October 13, 2018.
12. Pollin, R, Heintz, J, Arno, P et al. *In-Depth Analysis by Team of UMass Amherst Economists Shows Viability of Medicare for All*. Amherst, MA, November 30, 2018.
13. Meyer, H, Livingston, S, Dickson, V. CMS to allow states to define essential benefits. *Modern Healthcare*, October 29, 2017.
14. Verma, S, as quoted by Lighty, M. New Medicaid work requirements will deny more care. *Sanders Institute*, November 15, 2017.
15. Ross, C. Trump health official Seema Verma has a plan to slash Medicaid rolls. Here's how. *STAT*, October 26, 2017.
16. Galewitz, P. Evaluations of Medicaid experiments by state, CMS are weak. *Kaiser Health News*, February 23, 2018.
17. Healthcare-NOW! *Single –Payer Activist Guide to the Affordable Care Act.* Philadelphia, PA, 2013, p. 22.

18. Schulte, F. Audits of some Medicare Advantage plans reveal pervasive overcharging. *NPR Now* KPLU, August 29, 2016: 1.
19. Baker, S. The newest Medicare startup. *Axios Vitals*, October 24, 2017.
20. Himmelstein, DU, Woolhandler, S. The post-launch problem: The Affordable Care Act's persistently high administrative costs. *Health Affairs Blog*, May 27, 2017.
21. McCue, MJ, Bailit, MH. Assessing the financial health of Medicaid managed care plans and the quality of care they provide. New York. *The Commonwealth Fund*, June 15, 2011.
22. Terhune, C. Coverage denied; Medicaid patients suffer as layers of private companies profit. *Kaiser Health News*, January 3, 2019.)
23. Appleby, J. Trump administration loosens restrictions on short-term health plans. *Kaiser Health Plans*, August 1, 2018.
24. Appleby, J. Short-term health plans hold savings for consumers, profits for brokers and insurers. *Kaiser Health News*, December 21, 2018.
25. Appleby, J. Trump administration rule paves the way for association health plans. *Kaiser Health News*, January 4, 2018.
26. Cancryn, A. Trump promised them better, cheaper health care. It's not happening. *Politico*, July 19, 2018.
27. Mui, YQ. The shocking number of Americans who can't cover a $400 expense. *Washington Post on line*, May 25, 2016.
28. Terhune, C, Appleby, J. Companies behind health savings accounts could bank on big profits under GOP plan. *Kaiser Health News*, March 14, 2017.
29. Eskow, RJ. GOP 'Health' Bill: Death, disaster, and Gilded Age greed. *Common Dreams*, June 23, 2017.

CHAPTER 10

THE SHATTERED SAFETY NET
UNDER TRUMPCARE

As we saw in the last chapter, there is a long history of misguided information about health care which has blocked fundamental reform of U. S. health care for many years. All this is complicated by recurrent lies during the Trump administration. The goals of this chapter are two-fold: (1) to summarize the tax and budget cuts that have been enacted or proposed over the last two-plus years; and (2) to describe some of the ways that they have so adversely impacted a deteriorating safety net for much of our population.

Trump's Tax and Budget Cuts

The GOP has long waged war against "entitlement programs," especially Medicaid and Medicare, all of which was accelerated under the Trump administration. The onslaught against our safety net gained speed with the December 2017 tax cut bill, which repealed the individual mandate, led to an increase in the number of uninsured, and increased the federal deficit by an estimated $1.45 trillion. Since Medicare and Medicaid account for about 30 percent of the federal budget, they were increasingly targeted for future cutbacks under the guise of reducing the federal deficit. [1]

While media attention in October 2018 was focused on Senate hearings over Brett Kavanaugh's candidacy for the U. S. Supreme Court, the Republican-controlled Congress quietly passed another big tax handout to the wealthiest Americans. The corporate tax rate was reduced by 40 percent, leading not to trickle down job creation but to corporate stock buybacks and explosion of the federal deficit. [2]

The 2018 Bipartisan Budget Act passed by Congress in February 2018 increased military spending at the expense of big cuts in Medicare funding for long-term care. [3] Trump's budget proposal for 2019, also released in February 2018, called on lawmakers to gut the Supplemental Nutrition Assistance Program (SNAP or food stamps), eliminate the expansion of Medicaid under the ACA, transfer the rest of Medicaid into a system of capped payments to states, and expand requirements that low-income people work to qualify for assistance. [4] The new work requirements disregard the fact that most Medicaid recipients are already working and that most of those who are not are disabled. [5]

The Trump budget would slash budgets of Medicaid and Medicare by $1.3 trillion and $554 billion, respectively, reduce Social Security by $10 billion, cut funding for community health centers, as well as for subsidies that help more than four in five people to afford premiums in ACA marketplace plans. [6-8] These cuts became enmeshed in the ongoing heated debate within Congress over what would be enacted, and when, but can be summed up as a continued war against the poor and middle class.

In mid-March 2019, after his budget request of $5 billion for his wall at the southern border was rejected twice by Congress, Trump proposed a budget that would cut federal spending on Medicaid and Medicare by $1.4 trillion and more than $800 billion, respectively, over the coming decade. When legislators become aware of how block grants or severely capped federal payments of this magnitude will impact state budgets, this proposal is expected to receive a firestorm of resistance. [9]

Fortunately, these proposals are unlikely to become law with a Democrat-controlled House, but they reflect Trump's cruel and uncaring values. Wendell Potter, senior fellow on health care at the Center for Media and Democracy, and author of *Deadly Spin: An Insurance Company Insider Speaks Out On How Corporate PR Is Killing Health Care and Deceiving Americans*, made this observation:

> *It is obvious what he's attempting: Help the special interests loot our tax dollars, and then demand the most vulnerable Americans cover the difference.*[10]

As a result of these changes, inequality in wealth and income has become extreme as just a few billionaire family dynasties rig the U. S. economy. Median household wealth of Americans has declined since 1982 while the wealth of the Walton, Koch, and Mars families have grown by 6,000 percent. [11] The wealthiest 1 percent of American households own 40 percent of the country's wealth while the bottom 90 percent own just 20 percent. [12] Investors and money managers thrive on this widening wealth and income gap as health care stocks remain the best performer on the S & P 500. [13] The estate tax legislation being pushed by the Republican-controlled Senate threatens to worsen inequality even further, if passed. [14]

Jim Hightower is spot-on with this observation:

> *While Team Trump has been tirelessly saving corpo-*
> *rations from the "burden" of treating people with a modi-*
> *cum of fairness, it imposed truly onerous burdens on people*
> *needing the most help —including food, unemployment in-*
> *come, and health care. In April [2018], the president (who*
> *for years grabbed untold millions in public subsidies for his*
> *luxury resorts, casinos, condos, and hotels) signed an ex-*
> *ecutive order to "improve self sufficiency" by pushing ap-*
> *plicants for even basic allotments, such as $134 a month in*
> *food stamps, to first take a job—even at a sub-poverty pay,*
> *dead-end, dangerous job. By humiliating and stigmatizing*
> *the poor, such policies intend to kill support for even a bare-*
> *bones level of humane assistance.* [15]

Adverse Impacts on Deteriorating Safety Net

As we saw in Chapter 5 (Figure 5.2 on page 63), surprise medical bills are the biggest fear that Americans have, even more so than being able to afford such basic necessities as food, monthly utilities, or rental/mortgage payments. These unexpected medical bills are even worse for people who are sick or in poor health. [16]

Here are eight key areas that show the stark reality of the many circumstances that leave much of our population in dire straits every day.

1. Supplemental nutrition assistance program (SNAP)

This program, commonly known as food stamps, remains on the budget chopping list for conservative legislators, including work requirements to qualify for assistance. This is the size of the problem—41 million Americans are classified by the U. S. Department of Agriculture as being "food insecure," meaning that they are not sure where the next meals will come from. Family food insecurity exceeds 14 percent of those living in urban and rural areas. [17]

The farm bill passed by Congress in May 2018 took food stamps away from 2 million poor people, even though it failed to save money. [18] Food stamps are also not as beneficial as one might think, since they fail to cover the actual costs of a low-income meal in 99 percent of U. S. counties and the District of Columbia. [19]

2. Children

The Children's Health Insurance Program (CHIP) has been an essential part of our safety net for many years. It is mostly federally funded, and covers 9 million children from low-income families who earn too much to qualify for Medicaid. It too, however, has been on the chopping board for Republicans in Congress as another bloated entitlement program. Trump has wanted to cut $7 billion from the program, which remains vulnerable to future funding cuts by Congress. [20]

3. Women's health care

Despite being a majority of the population, women are more vulnerable to cuts in safety net and family planning programs than men. Compared to men, women are more likely to have lower wages and incomes, and to be the primary caretakers of their children. About 60 percent of low-wage workers are women, with almost 40 million on Medicaid. [21]

The U. S. has an unacceptably high maternal mortality rate (#46 in the world among developed nations and 7 times the rate for Finland). Between 700 and 900 women die every year from causes related to pregnancy or childbirth. In spite of this poor record, the

GOP and Trump administration continue their attacks on family planning programs such as Planned Parenthood. [22]

A new rule announced by DHHS in February 2019 stops federal funding under Title X to clinics that offer, promote or support abortion as a method of family planning. Targeting Planned Parenthood, the largest provider under the Title X family planning program, this rule is essentially a gag order prohibiting physicians or other health professionals in such clinics from discussing abortion with pregnant women, sharing information on that option, or making referrals for a safe and legal abortion. [23]

This family's story illustrates how wrong-headed these attacks are on programs that have been successful in protecting women from unwanted pregnancies and their risks.

Julie Liles, 31, and her 17 year-old daughter, Emily, attended a part of the Linking Families and Teens (LiFT) program. The mother-daughter pair found this program a very useful way to talk about relationships, love and sex through group discussions and role playing in a local high school. Despite the proven effectiveness of the federally funded Teen Pregnancy Prevention Program that involved more than a million teenagers across the country, this program was eliminated in July 2018 by the Trump administration. [24]

Trump's shutdown of the Teen Pregnancy Prevention Program flies in the face of experience documenting the effectiveness of family planning programs. As one example, a Colorado Family Planning Initiative started in 2009 achieved a 40 percent decline in teen births, 34 percent decline in teen abortions, and a saving of almost $6.00 in short-term Medicaid costs per dollar spent on the program. [25] Unfortunately, however, funding for this effective program was terminated.

4. Accountable care organizations (ACOs)

As networks of doctors and hospitals sharing medical and financial responsibility for groups of patients, accountable care organizations were initiated under the ACA in an attempt to save money and improve care. As a carrot-and-stick approach, the idea was that providers could make more money by keeping their patients healthier through ongoing coordination of care of a target population. ACOs therefore profit by spending less than they receive in their monthly allotment on patient care.

Not surprisingly, this has been a policy failure, since physicians and hospital systems can easily game the system by cherry picking patients and populations to be cared for. ACOs lose money by taking on the care of poorer and disadvantaged patients and populations, who are sicker and have worse outcomes because of socioeconomic determinants. As a result, physicians are incentivized to avoid these sicker patients, leaving them to what safety net they can find.

Despite their failure to save money or improve care, ACOs are still being promoted by the federal government, as this patient's story reflects.

Sandy Dowland, a 41 year-old mother of five who lives in a homeless shelter in Minneapolis, Minnesota, is fortunate to have Medicaid that has covered 10 E.R. visits in the last year, together with four hospitalizations. She has uncontrolled diabetes, high blood pressure, obesity, back pain, and major depression, and had a toe amputated during that time. But as the Minnesota Medicaid program is facing severe financial strains, it is exploring participating in an accountable care organization whereby they might hope to save money by keeping its spending within spending targets and potentially improving health outcomes and save money at the same time. [26]

5. Retirees and seniors

One used to be able to prepare for the future beyond retirement by purchasing long-term care insurance, but this industry is dying due to high and increasing costs of care for those who end up needing care in nursing homes, assisted living, or home care. Long-term care often costs more than $100,000 a year. Insurers are shying away from insuring these costs as they encounter a growing frequency and duration of claims. More than one-half of U. S. adults age 65 and older are expected to need nursing home or other care services in their later years, as shown in Figure 10.1.

What safety net can seniors count on in these new times when people are living longer and health care costs are unaffordable on fixed retirement incomes? Social Security provides 90 percent of income for one-third of the elderly and a majority of cash income for 61 percent of seniors. It continues under attack by Republicans who see its cuts as a way to reduce the federal deficit which their policies have exacerbated. [27] Meanwhile, public employers are increasingly cutting retiree health benefits and shifting to health reimbursement accounts (HRAs) that retirees can use as partial payment toward private insurance. [28]

FIGURE 10.1

LENGTH OF LONG TERM CARE NEEDED FOR U. S. SENIORS

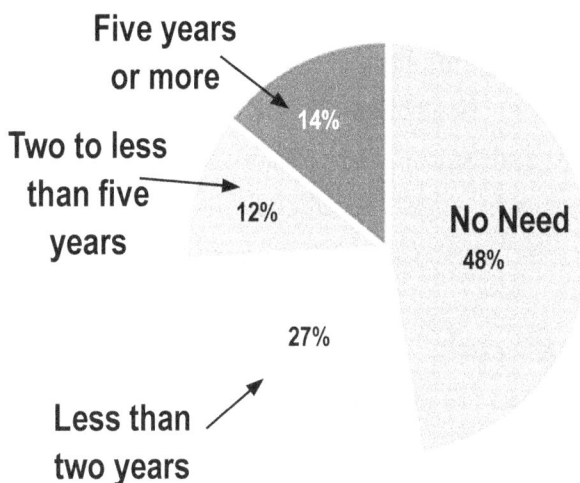

Five years
or more

14%

Two to less
than five
years

12%

No Need
48%

27%

Less than
two years

Source: Department of Health and Human Services

6. Mental illness

Mental health disorders affect one in five adults in this country, and are the leading cause of disability. But mental health care is poorly covered, if at all, by private insurers, and reimbursement for psychiatric services is so low that many health professionals avoid care of these patients. More than one-half of adults needing mental health care do not receive it in most states, together with up to one-third of children requiring such care. [29] As a result of limited or no access to mental health care, many mentally ill end up in jail, often without treatment. [30]

Almost one-half of the people held in more than 3,000 jails across the country have some kind of mental illness, more than one-quarter of which are severe. Their care is absent or poor in many cases, since that "care" has been increasingly contracted out to private for-profit companies that place profits over care. Now known as "correctional health care," this has become a $10 billion a year industry for companies that cut costs to raise profits and deny care to what is literally a captive market. Two of the largest companies, Corizon Health, based in Brentwood, Tennessee, and Wellpath, headquartered in Nashville, have been sued some 1,500 times over the last five years for alleged neglect, malpractice, and in dozens of cases, wrongful injury or death. [31]

7. Rural health care

Rural hospitals are the hub of accessible health care in most large rural areas, where they are usually the largest employer in the community but are under-reimbursed. They have been especially hard hit in recent years, leaving many patients without adequate care, especially for trauma, maternity care, and other urgently needed care. Almost 90 rural hospitals have closed since 2010, with many more at risk for closure. [32]

Here is one patient's story that illustrates the gravity of this problem.

A few hours after Twin Rivers Regional Medical Center closed in Kennett, Missouri, Kela Abernathy, 21, seven months pregnant, woke up in pain with early labor at 4:30 a.m. The only hospital in town, it used to be just around the corner, but had been closed on short notice by Community Health Systems, a publicly traded, for-profit company. The 116-bed hospital had been a lifeline for the county's 32,000 people, with about 22,000 E. R. visits and 400 obstetric deliveries a year. At the time of its closure, the hospital's CEO could only say that this was "the most sustainable plan for the future." The local message was "Hospital closed. Call 911 for emergencies."

Kela, her 2-year old son, and mother grabbed a few bags, jumped into their car, and raced down dark country roads across southeast Missouri seeking the nearest care. The closest hospital was 20 miles away in Hayti, but its obstetric unit had been closed four years earlier and an ambulance was not available, leaving the nearest obstetric care 80 miles away at St. Francis Medical Center in Cape Girardeau. After a four-hour trip, they reached that hospital in time to have an emergency caesarian section for twins, Kaleb at 3 pounds 6 ounces and Kylynn at 2 pounds 12 ounces. The infants were healthy, but would need many weeks of close care at the hospital, with Kela having to make regular 200-mile round trips to the hospital to see them. [33]

This has become a common story in rural America as rural hospitals are being financially battered by cuts in public safety net programs, shortages of physicians and nurses, and increasing debt, especially in states that did not expand Medicaid under the ACA.

Other parts of the crisis in rural health care are the closure of nursing homes and pharmacies in rural areas. More than 440 rural nursing homes have closed or merged over the last decade, leaving their communities without such facilities. [34] Meanwhile, over 600 rural communities lost their only local pharmacy over the last 15 years, their only source of available prescription medications on a timely basis. Their closure is in large part due to exploitive and little known pricing policies of profiteering pharmacy benefit managers (PBMs), which "manage" some 90 percent of prescription drug sales in the country, raise costs to patients, and pay rural pharmacies amounts way below their acquisition costs. [35]

8. Immigrant care

There has long been a misguided bias among conservatives in this country that immigrants place a heavy burden on our health care system and don't pay their way. However, a recent study found that notion to be completely false. Immigrants, both documented and undocumented, accounted for 12.6 percent of premiums paid to private insurers in 2014, but used only 9.1 percent of insurer expenditures. Instead of being a burden, immigrants subsidized our system for U. S. born beneficiaries by $174.4 billion between 2008 and 2014. [36]

The Trump administration, however, continues this now discredited bias and comes down hard on immigrants with his anti-immigrant policies that are an integral part of his nationalistic "Make America Great" slogan. Families have been separated under his zero-tolerance policy, with thousands of children still separated from their parents today. Exact numbers and the whereabouts of the children are not available.

Health care for migrants at the southern border is typically absent or inadequate, as this child's story illustrates.

> *Rosa Maria Hernandez, a ten-year old girl with cerebral palsy, was enroute to a hospital 80 miles away for emergency gallbladder surgery when the ambulance carrying her was stopped at an immigration checkpoint. Instead of allowing the ambulance to proceed, Border Patrol followed her to the hospital, maintained surveillance throughout the procedure, and camped outside her room until she was discharged. She was then taken back into custody and referred to the Office of Refugee Resettlement, separating her from her parents and family members. Only national outrage gained her eventual release. The Department of Homeland Security saw no problem with this course of action. The ACLU filed suit in this matter, eventually securing her release.* [37]

Figure 10.2 illustrates the moral vacuum of the Trump administration's zero-tolerance policy. Management of the federal government's detention centers along our southern border are becoming a growing line of business for for-profit private companies that charge $750 a day to house migrant children, three times the actual cost, with taxpayers paying for these profits. [38]

FIGURE 10.2

Chaos for Migrants at the Border

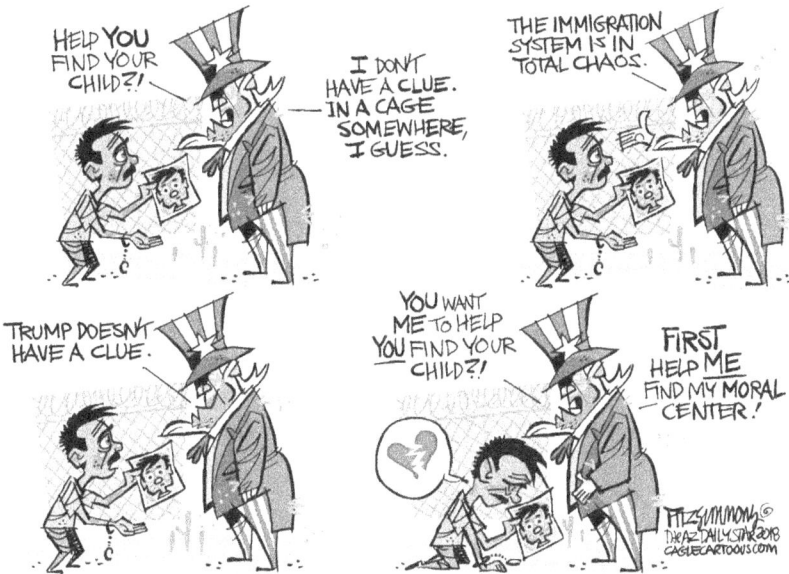

Source: Courtesy of Fitzimmons @ the *AZ Daily Star*, 2018

Continuing the Trump administration's hostility to immigrants, the Department of Homeland Security released a proposed rule in September 2018 that any immigrant who is likely to use or who has already used Medicaid, food stamps, public housing, a rent voucher, or other cash assistance, could be barred from the country or barred from getting permanent resident status. This rule would redefine self-sufficiency in an effort to admit only those who will never need a public safety net. As Bryce Covert wrote in an Op-Ed for the *The Washington Post*:

> *This redefinition of self-sufficiency ignores the way that most people use these programs. Even people with jobs often cycle on and off assistance as work comes and goes, or to plug the gaps when it just doesn't pay enough. These programs allow people to remain healthy and solvent—supporting their independence. This rule therefore hurts everyone, not just immigrants, by stigmatizing the safety net funded by all of us to help people survive when they fall on hard times.[39]*

Conclusion

Unfortunately, the above patient stories are all too common, and worse, they are getting even more common. The GOP tax cuts and policies of the Trump administration have ruptured whatever safety net we used to have. Altogether, they are un-American in this country which supposedly has higher values.

These policies are also a complete giveaway to the wealthy as inequality in our society grows without restraints. An entire new corporate industry has also emerged to handle the complex and changing eligibility for means-tested programs such as Medicaid and CHIP, including managing the work requirements of Medicaid. Subcontracting for the minutiae of public-benefit paperwork and accounting has attracted such corporate behemoths as Hewlett-Packard and IBM. Maximus is another new entrant to this lucrative business, now involved in ongoing case management of about 59 percent of Medicaid clients in 41 states across the country. Richard Montoni, its CEO, took in $9.45 million in executive compensation in 2017. [40]

We can hope that the new 116th Democratic-controlled House of Representatives can reverse these disastrous cuts in our safety net and more effectively oppose the greed from the wealthy and corporate interests through tax reform. We can also hope that the final 2020 Democratic candidate for the presidency, together with the Democratic platform, can strongly advocate for real health care reform—Medicare for All, which can overnight provide universal access to affordable health care for all U. S. residents—the ultimate safety net.

How can we tolerate the loss of a safety net for much of our population? Aren't we a better country than this? In the next and last two chapters, we will explore and try to answer these questions.

References

1. Blumenthal, D. How the new U. S. tax plan will affect health care. *Harvard Business Review*, December 19, 2017.
2. Clemente, F. Under cover of Kavanaugh, Republicans passed huge tax cuts for the wealthy. *The Progressive Populist*, November 1, 2018.
3. Lawson, A. Trump's budget calls for $1.8 trillion in cuts to earned benefits. *Social Security Works*, February 12, 2018.
4. Jan, T, Dewey, C, Goldstein, A et al. Trump wants to overhaul America's safety net with giant cuts to housing, food stamps, and health care. *The Washington Post*, February 12, 2018.
5. Washington Post Staff. What Trump proposed cutting in his 2019 budget. *The Washington Post*, February 16, 2018.
6. Williams, B. Stop cheering the budget deal. It's a blow to long-term care and the safety net. *USA Today*, February 15, 2018.
7. Tracy, J, Dewey, C, Goldstein, A et al. Trump wants to overhaul America's safety net with giant cuts to housing, food stamps and health care. *The Washington Post*, February 12, 2018.
8. Garfield, R, Rudowitz, R, Damico, A. Understanding the intersection of Medicaid and work. *Kaiser Family Foundation*, January 5, 2018.

9. Pear, R. Congress warns against Medicaid cuts: 'You just wait for the firestorm.' *New York Times*, March 12, 2019.
10. Potter, W. Trump's greedy 2019 budget goes nuclear on Medicare and Medicaid. *Common Dreams*, March 13, 2019.
11. Johnson, J. A handful of billionaire families grab nation's wealth for themselves, new report details how dynasties rig U. S. economy. *Common Dreams*, October 30, 2018.
12. Ingraham, C. The richest 1 percent now owns more of the country's wealth than at any time in the past 50 years. *The Washington Post*, December 6, 2017.
13. Wursthorn, M. Health care stocks take rally's lead. *Wall Street Journal*, September 26, 2018: B 15.
14. Johnson, J. 'Greed has no limit for GOP': McConnell estate tax repeal would hand tens of billions to Walton and Koch families. *Common Dreams*, January 29, 2019.
15. Hightower, J. Trump's privatizers are running amuk. *The Hightower Lowdown*, September 2018.
16. Altman, D. It's not just the uninsured—it's also the cost of health care. *Axios*, August 20, 2018.
17. Alterman, E. Hungry and invisible. *The Nation*, November 13, 2017.
18. Rampell, C. Congress takes food from 2 million poor people—and doesn't even save money. *The Washington Post*, May 17, 2018.
19. Waxman, E. How far do SNAP benefits fall short of covering the cost of a meal? *Urban Institute*, February 22, 2018.
20. Galewitz, P. 4 takeaways from Trump's plan to rescind CHIP funding. *Kaiser Health News*, May 8, 2018.
21. Bernstein, J, Katch, H. Cutting support for economically vulnerable women is no way to celebrate Mother's Day. *The Washington Post*, May 11, 2018.
22. West, E. Why single-payer is a feminist issue. *Truthout*, January 21, 2018.
23. Gallegos, A. Trump bars abortion referrals from family planning program. MDedge *ObGyn*, February 22, 2019.
24. Kodjak, A. Trump administration sued over ending funding of teen pregnancy programs. *NPR*, February 15, 2018.
25. Pollitt, K. Magic-bullet birth control? *The Nation*, June 8, 2015, p. 10.
26. Galewitz, P. As Medicaid costs soar, states try a new approach. *Kaiser Health News*, June 15, 2018.
27. vanden Heuvel, K. Voters must catch on to Republicans' con on health care. *The Washington Post*, October 24, 2018.
28. Farmer, L. As retiree health care costs soar, public employers turn to private insurers. *Governing*, January 9, 2019.
29. Radley, DC, McCarthy, D, Hayes, SL. 2018 Scorecard on State Health

System Performance. New York. *The Commonwealth Fund.*

30. Gorman, A. Use of psychiatric drugs soars in California jails. *Kaiser Health News*, May 8, 2018.

31. Coll, S. The jail health-care crisis. *The New Yorker,* March 4, 2019.

32. Frakt, A. A sense of alarm as rural hospitals keep closing. *New York Times*, October 29, 2018.

33. Healy, J. It's 4 a.m. The baby's coming. But the hospital is 100 miles away. *New York Times*, July 17, 2018.

34. Healy, J. Nursing homes are closing across rural America, scattering residents. *New York Times*, March 4, 2019.

35. Langreth, R, Ingold, D, Gu, J. Secret drug pricing system middlemen use to rake in millions. *Bloomberg*, September 11, 2018.

36. Zallman, L, Woolhandler, D. Touw, S et al. Immigrants pay more in private insurance premiums than they receive in benefits. *Health Affairs* 37 (10): 1663-1668.

37. ACLU. Release 10-year old Rosa Maria. American Civil Liberties Union, October 31, 2017.

38. Torbati, Y, Cooke, K. First stop for migrant kids: For-profit detention center. *Politicus USA*, February 15, 2019 by Reuters.

39. Covert, B. Trump wants to turn the safety net into a trap. *New York Times*, October 1, 2018.

40. McMillan, T. How one company is making millions off Trump's war on the poor. *Mother Jones*, January/February, 2019.

PART III

CAN U. S. HEALTH CARE BE REFORMED IN THE PUBLIC INTEREST?

Over the years I have aligned myself with unpopular causes. I have worked to replace the worship of the market with concern for the common good, social justice and tolerance. Over time the American people usually do the right thing, and I am confident they will see that national health insurance is no longer the best solution, it is the only solution.

— Quentin Young, M. D., internist, former chairman of medicine at Cook County Hospital in Chicago, long-time political activist for social justice, and author of *Everybody In, Nobody Out: Memoirs of a Rebel Without a Pause.*

The great corporations . . . are the creatures of the State, and the State has not only the right to control them, but it is duty-bound to control them wherever the need of control is shown.

—President Theodore Roosevelt, 1902.

CHAPTER 11

IS HEALTH CARE A RIGHT IN A CIVILIZED SOCIETY?

You might think this question would be a no-brainer, but you would be wrong. After 70 years, it remains controversial in this country, and the U. S. continues as an outlier in the world community of advanced countries.

This chapter has two goals: (1) to bring an historical perspective to how health care as a human right has been dealt with in other advanced countries compared to this country; and (2) to present the case for its acceptance in the U.S. for medical, public health, economic, social, moral, and political reasons.

Health Care as a Human Right: An Historical Perspective

International organizations have recognized health care as a human right all the way back to 1948, when the General Assembly of the United Nations adopted the Universal Declaration of Human Rights. The right to health care was later adopted, also, by the World Health Organization (WHO) in its Declaration on the Rights of Patients. [1] The issue soon became enmeshed in the debate over universal access to health care, which in subsequent years led to systems of universal coverage in almost all advanced countries around the world, but not here.

Efforts to establish universal coverage through National Health Insurance (NHI) go back farther in this country than most people realize, always with lack of success. It was first brought into the public debate in 1912 when Theodore Roosevelt made it a platform plank for the Progressive Party. [2] The preceding 30 years had seen many European countries adopt one or another form of universal coverage, usually as sickness insurance, with Germany the first in 1883. [3]

Congress held hearings in 1916 on a federal plan to provide disability and sickness benefits as momentum was gathering toward some sort of national plan. Remarkably, the American Medical Association (AMA) at first adopted this supportive resolution in 1917 as recommended by its social insurance committee:

The time is present when the profession should study earnestly to solve the questions of medical care that will arise under various forms of social insurance. Blind opposition, indignant repudiation, bitter denunciation of these laws is worse than useless; it leads nowhere and it leaves the profession in a position of helplessness as the rising tide of social development sweeps over it. [4]

That recommendation did not last long after strong opposition came back from the AMA's state chapters, and that kind of resistance has continued to this day.

In the late 1920s, the Committee on the Costs of Medical Care (CCMC) was formed, an influential independent commission with private funding that included physicians, public health professionals, and economists. As the Great Depression enveloped the country, the CCMC led the charge toward NHI. [5] A landmark report by another commission, the Committee on Economic Security (which led to the Social Security Act of 1935), also endorsed NHI. Largely due to consolidated opposition from the AMA, however, President Franklin D. Roosevelt (FDR) dropped NHI from the Social Security Act to ensure its passage. At the same time, an alternative to compulsory health insurance was being promoted by a newly founded private company, Blue Cross, whose leaders argued that:

> *Blue Cross coverage would eliminate the demand for compulsory health insurance and stop the reintroduction of vicious sociological bills into the state legislature year after year—Blue Cross Plans are a distinctly American institution, a unique combination of individual initiative and social responsibility. They perform a public service without public compulsion.* [6]

Although FDR postponed NHI in 1935, he did not abandon it, and added the issue to his legislative agenda in the 1944 State of the Union address. He asked Congress for "an economic bill of rights," to include a plan for adequate medical care. [7] He died in 1945 before he could see his proposal through, but his successor, President Harry Truman proposed a comprehensive NHI plan in 1946, to be administered through the Social Security system. Again, however, opposing interests defeated the bill by lobbying a Republican-controlled Congress against it and stoking the public's fears of "socialism." [8] The AMA lobbied for voluntary health insurance and indigent care services, claiming that NHI would "turn physicians into slaves. [9]

All was quiet on the NHI front during the 1950s and 1960s, but health insurance for the elderly was a major issue during the presidential elections of 1960 and 1964. How the U. S. should interpret and apply the right to health care was a continuing divisive issue across the political spectrum, with liberals supporting this right and conservatives countering that it was a "qualified right granted patients but modified by the available resources within the health care system and the rights of physicians to control the practice of their professions." [10]

The passage of Medicare in 1965 ended a long journey seeking health insurance for older Americans through the administrations of FDR, Truman, Eisenhower, Kennedy, and Johnson. A 1965 Gallup poll found that 61 percent of respondents supported this compulsory health insurance plan for the elderly based on the concept of social insurance. [11] Still, the AMA maintained its stance against Medicare, regarding it as "big government intruding into private markets and a first step toward government control of health care." A potential legislative stalemate was avoided, however, by the concurrent passage of Medicaid, which was largely the work of opponents to Medicare. [12]

The Nixon administration in 1970 found itself dealing with numerous liberal initiatives from a Democrat-controlled Congress. Sen. Ted Kennedy proposed a single-payer NHI plan on this basis:

Health care is not just another commodity. It is not a gift to be rationed based on the ability to pay. It is time to make universal health insurance a national priority, so that the basic right to health care can finally become a reality for every American.

It was still not to be, however, as Nixon was besieged by the Watergate scandal and Vietnam, and it was not possible to forge bipartisan support for NHI.

The 1980s and early 1990s were marked by increasing competition and consolidation within the medical-industrial complex. Managed care by private companies was taking center stage, and Blue Cross plans were increasingly converting to for-profit status in a corporatized marketplace. Health care reform was a big issue during the 1992 elections. Rep. Jim McDermott (D. WA) introduced a single-payer proposal in the House (H.R. 1200). Although it had strong grassroots support, attracted the largest number of supporters in Congress of any of the competing proposals and was the only one of five proposals to pass out of committee, it was effectively opposed by its opponents and marginalized by the media.[13] The competing 1,342 page Clinton Health Plan was byzantine in its complexity and was dead on arrival in Congress. Its fatal flaw was seen as trying to combine employer mandates (which attracted health interests and repelled many employers) and cost controls (which attracted employers and repelled health interests)![14]

Opposition by corporate stakeholders and the AMA to any form of NHI continued throughout the early 2000s. In 2003, Rep. John Conyers (D. MI) introduced his Expanded and Improved Medicare for All bill as H.R. 676 in the House, where it resided without action in succeeding Congresses. The next major proposal for NHI was brought forward by Sen. Bernie Sanders during the 2016 elections as S. 1804 in the Senate. These two bills will be on center stage during the 2020 election campaigns, with Rep. Pramila Jayapal (D. WA) and Rep. Debbie Dingman (D. MI) cosponsors of the new Medicare for All Act of 2019 (H.R. 1384).

The Case for Health Care as a Human Right

If we step back and ask ourselves who is our health care system for, we should readily come up with the obvious—for patients and their families, not for corporate interests sucking our wallets empty as so many millions of Americans delay or go without needed care, or have to declare bankruptcy because of the high costs of essential care. Equally obvious from the above history, corporate stakeholders and their allies, including the private insurance industry and Big PhRMA, investors and Wall Street, have so far defeated any effort toward a national health insurance plan serving our entire population.

We can make an overwhelming case for finally enacting NHI in this country, based on these arguments.

Medical

As previous chapters have fully documented, we have an accelerating crisis in U. S. health care, with restricted access to care, unaffordable costs, unacceptable outcomes of care, and a failing and unsustainable private health insurance industry that is profiteering off taxpayer dollars.

America today has a two-tier health care system, with a growing divide between the haves and have-nots. As one example, urgent care centers are absent in low-income neighborhoods in the Boston area, with four in the higher-income Cambridge. As Joan Vennochi asks in an Op-Ed for the *Boston Globe*: "Should it be OK to make it harder for poor people to qualify for urgent care? Are the poor so different from the rest of us that they should have fewer health care options? We all get sick." [15]

Public health

The goal of public health is "to secure health and promote wellness for both individuals and communities, by addressing societal, environmental, and individual determinants of health." [16] Arguably, many of the major improvements in the health of our population have been accomplished more through public health approaches than by individual-based health care.

In the 1990s, these ten areas gained the most important advances in population health, all of which are equally relevant today:

1. Vaccination
2. Motor vehicle safety
3. Safer workplaces
4. Control of infectious diseases
5. Decline in deaths from coronary heart disease and stroke
6. Safer and healthier foods
7. Healthier mothers and babies
8. Family planning
9. Fluoridation of drinking water
10. Recognition of tobacco use as a health hazard. [17]

Vaccination makes the point clearly, since the higher the vaccination rates are across the population, the safer we all are in being protected from infectious diseases.

Economic

Aside from the public who will be best served with universal coverage under NHI, providers in today's health care system will also do well. Hospitals, clinics, nursing homes, and other facilities will gain stability through annual global budgets. Mental health care and public health will be adequately funded for the first time, together with other safety net facilities and programs. All those involved in rural health care will find themselves in a stabilized and predictable environment.

Physicians and other health professionals will remain in private practice and be well compensated through negotiated fees. Employers will be relieved of their growing burden of providing employer sponsored health insurance to their employees, and will be better able to compete in global markets. Despite new negotiated prices, pharmaceutical and medical device companies will do well the old fashioned way by competing on the basis of the efficacy and quality of their products in one big market through bulk purchasing under NHI.

Social

Social security and traditional Medicare are good examples of social insurance that bring us together. As future beneficiaries, we pay into them over the years. They have become fundamental parts of the social fabric of this country, as will happen if we all pay toward Medicare for All through progressive taxes. As Theodore Marmor, Jerry Mashaw, and John Pakutka state in their important 2014 book, *Social Insurance: America's Neglected Heritage and Contested Future*:

> *The core features of social insurance programs are economically sensible and socially legitimate and thus glue that holds an individualistic polity together and that make the economic risks of a market economy tolerable.* [18]

We have only to look north of our border to better understand the cohesive impact of NHI. Tommy Douglas, acclaimed across the country as the father of universal health care in Canada, is regarded as a national hero. Canadians highly value and support their single-payer health care, with freedom of choice and unimpeded access to needed health care without co-payments. They regard their health care as a basic right and a cornerstone of their country's social structure.

Moral

Whether we recognize it or not, we are all in the same boat. All of us will get sick and need access to necessary care at some points in our lives, often on an urgent or emergency basis. Health care is an essential need for both individuals and populations, and is more available if not treated as a commodity for sale in a for-profit marketplace that shuns people who can't pay up front. Drs. David Himmelstein and Steffie Woolhandler, professors of public health at the City University of New York, make this persuasive point:

> *In our society, some aspects of life are off-limits to commerce. We prohibit the selling of children and the buying of wives, juries, and kidneys. Tainted blood is an inevitable consequence of paying blood donors; even sophisticated laboratory tests cannot compensate for blood that is sold rather than given as a gift. Like blood, health care is too precious, intimate, and corruptible to entrust to the market.* [19]

Jonas Salk, who developed the first effective vaccine for polio in the 1950s, gave us a classic example of moral leadership in his answer to Edward R. Murrow's question about who would own the patent:

The American people, I guess. Could you patent the sun? [20]

Larry Churchill, Ph.D., an ethicist at the University of Notre Dame, brings us this useful insight on the role and limits of health care as a human right:

> *There is a moral right to health care, but not of the sort often claimed. It is a right grounded not in purchasing power, merit, or social worth, but in human need. The right to health care finds its rationale in a social concept of the self, in a sense of common humanity, and in a knowledge of common vulnerability to disease and death. . . . A right to health care based on need means a right to equitable access based on need alone to all effective care society can reasonably afford.. . . . A right to health care is not a license to demand care. It is not a right to the very best available, or even to all one may need. Some very pressing health needs may have to be neglected because meeting them would be unreasonable in the light of other health needs or social priorities.* [21]

Ban Ki-moon, former Secretary-General of the United Nations from 2007 through 2016, has denounced U. S. health care as unethical, politically wrong, and morally wrong. He accuses "the powerful interests of pharmaceutical companies, hospitals and doctors as inhibiting the American government from moving toward universal health care." [22]

Political

Marmor and his colleagues have observed how stabilizing and cohesive social insurance is in a society, and they have this to add:

> *Social insurance programs* [such as traditional Medicare and NHI] *engage most of the electorate precisely because they cover common risks and insure most of the population.*

166

And because practically everyone is both a contributor and a potential beneficiary, the politics of social insurance tends to be of the "us-us" rather than "us-them" form. Each individual's sense of earned entitlement or deservingness makes reneging on promises in social insurance programs politically costly. [23]

Conclusion

If we can make our democracy work, with 70 percent of Americans supporting NHI, together with 80-plus percent of Democrats and a Democrat-controlled House of Representatives, the 2020 elections may be the best chance in many years to achieve NHI. In the next and last chapter, we will examine what the odds are in this new political environment.

References

1. Carmi, A. On patients' rights. *Med. Law*, 1991; 10 (1): 77-81.
2. Somers, AR, Somers, HM. *Health and Health Care: Policies in Perspective.* Germantown, MD; *Aspen Systems Corp.*,1977: 179-180.
3. Starr, P. *The Social Transformation of American Medicine.* New York. *Basic Books*, 1982.
4. Burrow, JG. *AMA: Voice of American Medicine.* Baltimore: *Johns Hopkins Press*, 1963: 144.
5. Davis, MM. The American approach to health insurance. *Milbank Q*, July 12, 1934: 214-215.
6. Rothman, DJ. The public presentation of Blue Cross, 1935-1965. *J Health Polit Policy Law*, 1991: 16 (4): 671-693.
7. Ibid # 2.
8. Thai, KV, Qiao, Y, McManus, SM. National health care reform failure: The political economy perspective. *J Health Hum Serv Adm.* Fall 1998; 21 (2): 236-259.
9. Poen, M. *Harry S. Truman versus the Medical Lobby: The Genesis of Medicare.* Columbia; University of Missouri Press, 1979: 85-86.

10. Kaufmann, CL. The right to health care: Some cross-national comparisons and U. S. trends in policy. *Soc. Sci. Med.* 1981; 15(4): 157-162.
11. Marmor, TR. *The Politics of Medicare.* Third edition. Hawthorne, NY. *Aldine de Gruyter, Inc.* 2000, xxiv-xxv.
12. Marmor, TR, Mashaw, JL, Pakutka, J. *Social Insurance: America's Neglected Heritage and Contested Future.* Washington, D.C. *Sage Copress*, 2014, 61.
13. Brundin, J. How the U. S. press covers the Canadian health care system. *Intl J Health Serv* 1993; 23(2): 275-277.
14. Gordon, C. The Clinton Health Care Plan: Dead on Arrival. Westfield, NJ. *Open Magazine Pamphlet Series*, 1995.
15. Vennochi, J. We all get sick. It shouldn't be harder for poor people to have access to urgent care centers. *Boston Globe*, January 14, 2019.
16. The Institute for the Future. *Health and Health Care 2010: The Forecast, the Challenge.* San Francisco. *Jossey-Bass*, 2000.
17. Centers for Disease Control and Prevention. Ten great public health achievements—United States, 1990-1999. *MMWR Morb Mortal Wkly Rep.* 1999; 48: 241-243.
18. Ibid # 12, p. 217.
19. Woolhandler, S, Himmelstein, DU. When money is the mission: the high costs of investor-owned care. *N Engl J Med* 1999; 341; 444-446.
20. Smith, J. *Patenting the Sun: Polio and the Salk vaccine.* New York. *William Morrow*, 1990, p. 159.
21. Churchill, LR. *Rationing Health Care in America: Perceptions and Principles of Justice.* Notre Dame, IN. *University of Notre Dame*, 1987: 90-91, 94-96.
22. Ki-moon, B, as quoted by Glenza, J. Ex-UN chief Ban Ki-moon says U. S. health care system is 'morally wrong.' *The Guardian*, September 25, 2018.
23. Ibid # 2, p.219-220,

CHAPTER 12

HOW U. S. HEALTH CARE
CAN BE REFORMED

Now that we have completed our journey across the profit-driven corporate medical-industrial complex, the big question remains: can our very sick health care system be reformed in the public interest? The answer, of course, is YES, but requires education of policymakers, legislators and the public, plus political will.

This final chapter has two goals: (1) to discuss the major elements required to reform U. S. health care on an affordable and sustainable basis for the common good; and (2) to describe the current political landscape of the battleground that must be won for this to happen.

Key Elements of Health Care Reform
1. Financing reform from multi-payer to single-payer

The most important reform of all is to change how we finance health care. Our present mostly private, multi-payer system is overly complex, bureaucratic, wasteful, and unsustainable as it profits on the backs of patients, their families, and taxpayers.

There are now two single-payer Medicare for All bills in the 116th session of Congress, the Medicare for All Act of 2019 (H. R. 1384 in the House), with Rep. Pramila Jayapal (D. WA) and Rep. Debbie Dingell (D. MI) the lead sponsors), and S-1804, sponsored by Sen. Bernie Sanders (I-VT) in the Senate. The House bill was released on February 27, 2019, with 107 co-sponsors, and has already been cleared for hearings by several committees. These are its main provisions:

- Creates a new system of national health insurance (NHI), with equity for all based on medical need, and on the principle that health care is a human right, not a privilege based on ability to pay.
- Universal access to health care for all U. S. residents, with free choice of providers and hospital anywhere in the country without restrictive networks.
- Covers all medically necessary care, including ambulatory care; hospitalization and doctor visits; laboratory and diagnostic services; dental, vision, and hearing care; prescription drugs; reproductive health, including abortion; maternity and newborn care; mental health services including substance abuse treatment; and long-term care services and supports.
- Eliminates all patient cost-sharing such as co-pays, deductibles, and premiums.
- Eliminates pre-authorizations or other restrictions now imposed by private insurers.
- Pays institutions such as hospitals and nursing homes via lump sum annual operating budgets to provide covered items and services.
- Pharmaceutical reform, including negotiated drug prices.
- Administrative simplification with efficiencies and cost containment through large-scale cost controls, including (a) negotiated fee schedules for physicians and other health professionals, who will remain in private practice;

(b) global budgeting of individual hospitals and other facilities; and (c) bulk purchasing of drugs and medical devices giving consideration to their comparative clinical and cost effectiveness.

- Elimination of the private health insurance industry, with its large administrative overhead and profiteering, and employer-sponsored health insurance.
- Establishes an Office of Primary Health Care, tasked with developing and coordinating national goals related to education of health care professionals and expanding the number of primary care practitioners.
- Shared risk for the costs of illness and accidents across the entire population of 326 million.

These are the main provisions of H. R. 1384 which are different from the earlier Conyers bill in the House (H. R. 676):

- Adds more comprehensive benefits, including dental, vision, prescription drugs; approved dietary and nutritional therapies; podiatric care; emergency services and transportation; early and periodic screening, diagnostic, and treatment services; necessary transportation for health care services for persons with disabilities or who may qualify as low income; and improved long-term services and supports.
- Lengthens transition period from one to two years; one year after enacted, U. S. residents over age 55 and under 19 will be covered.
- Overrides the Hyde amendment that bans public funding of abortion.
- Allows override of drug patents when drug companies demand extortionate prices.

- Preserves separate Veterans Administration and Indian Health Service.
- Provides regional funding for rural and urban areas that are medically underserved.
- Allocates 1 percent of budget for the first five years to assistance and retraining for workers displaced by elimination of the private health insurance industry.

The Senate bill, S-1804, differs from the new House bill, H.R. 1384, in these respects:

- Retains for-profit, investor owner ownership of facilities without global budgets.
- Maintains current Medicare payment models, resulting in higher costs.
- Does not cover long-term services except by preserving Medicaid for that purpose, as well as supports for people with disabilities and older persons.
- Includes co-pays for prescription drugs, with a cap of $200 per year for each person enrolled in the program.
- Four-year transition period.

Both the House bill and the Senate bill will create a new system of national health insurance (NHI) which will share risk for health care costs across the largest possible risk pool. Since we know that 20 percent of the population accounts for about 80 percent of all health care spending—the "20-80 rule"—this is the most efficient way to spread risk for the costs of health care. [1] As a result, private insurers can no longer segment risk pools in their favor by selecting healthier enrollees and shifting sicker patients to public programs.

2. Paying for Medicare for All with savings and progressive taxation.

Supporters of H. R. 1384 have so far been silent on how to finance Medicare for All, and the Congressional Budget Office is in the process of reviewing the proposal. We do, however, have an excellent recent study, released on November 30, 2018 by the Political Economy Research Institute (PERI) at the University of Massachusetts-Amherst, which found that single-payer Expanded and Improved Medicare for All will save the U. S. $5.1 trillion over a decade through savings from our market-based, multi-payer system. That study estimates that total annual health care spending in this country will increase over a decade from $3.2 trillion to $3.6 trillion as millions of people get care that they previously had to forgo, but that number will be reduced by big savings in administrative, pharmaceutical, and provider payment spending. [2,3]

The PERI study set out this approach for progressive taxes:
1. Business premiums 8 percent below what a business now spends on health care.
2. 3.75 percent sales tax on non-essential goods.
3. Recurring tax of 0.36 percent on all wealth over $1 million.
4. Taxing long-term capital gains as regular income.

Based on this approach, the PERI study projects that middle-class Americans will see savings of up to 14 percent, while high-income Americans will have only a small increase in their total health care spending. (Figure 12.1) [4]

FIGURE 12.1

Percent Change in Health Care Spending Under Medicare for All by Income Level and Insurance Status, 2016

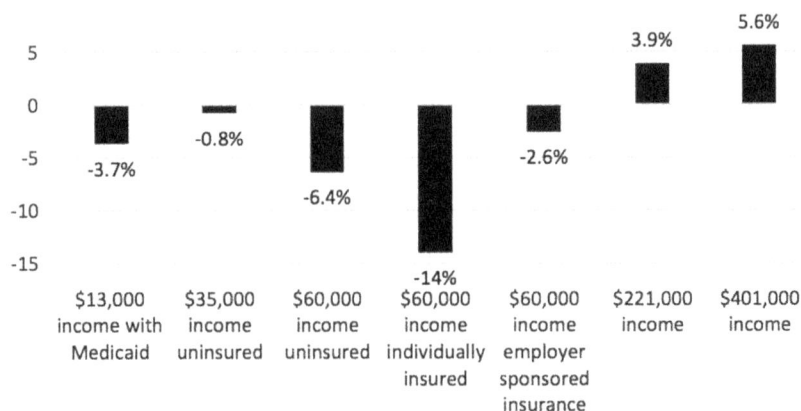

Sources: 2016 American Community Survey, the Consumer Expenditure Survey, and others.

3. Elimination of the private health insurance industry

This is a sine qua non for any substantive health care reform. Over the last four decades, the private health insurance industry has placed profits ahead of service and has abused the public trust. With its top priority being to maximize revenue for CEOs and shareholders, insurers leave markets on short notice when profits do not meet their expectations. The ACA did nothing to reverse this behavior as the industry continues to game the system at patients' expense, such as through higher cost-sharing, more restrictive networks, deceptive marketing practices, and limited drug formularies.

Since the advent of managed care in the late 1980s and 1990s, private insurers have developed bloated bureaucracies in order to set limits on referrals and hospitalizations, deny services, and dis-enroll sick enrollees. Between 2000 and 2005, its workforce grew by one-third, even as the insurance market declined by one percent. [5] The administrative overhead and profits of private insurers run between 18 and 20 percent, compared to 2.5 percent for traditional Medicare. [6] Over the last two years under the Trump administration, this bureaucracy has grown even larger, especially as more responsibility for Medicaid shifts to the states under relaxed federal rules. Overpayments are widespread for both privatized Medicare and Medicaid. Unnecessary or duplicative payments to providers in private Medicaid plans are common in more than 30 states. [7]

The private health insurance industry has not, and cannot contain health care costs. Traditional public Medicare gives us a good example of effective cost containment. Over the last 20 years, Medicare's cumulative costs declined by almost 2 percent while those of private insurance grew by more than 16 percent. (Figure 12.2) [8] Comparing costs of inpatient hospital stays over 20 years, as another example, traditional Medicare kept costs even while private insurers saw an increase of more than 65 percent. (Figure 12.3) [9]

The federal government now pays about 60 percent of total health care costs in this country, a much higher figure than most taxpayers realize. Much of this has been ongoing subsidies of the private health insurance industry, which receives $685 billion in government subsidies each year; the CBO projects this number to double in another ten years. [10]

We, including the public, policymakers, and legislators, have

FIGURE 12.2

PERCENTAGE CHANGE IN HEALTH CARE COSTS FOR ENROLLEES IN PRIVATE INSURANCE VS. MEDICARE, 2009 - 2016

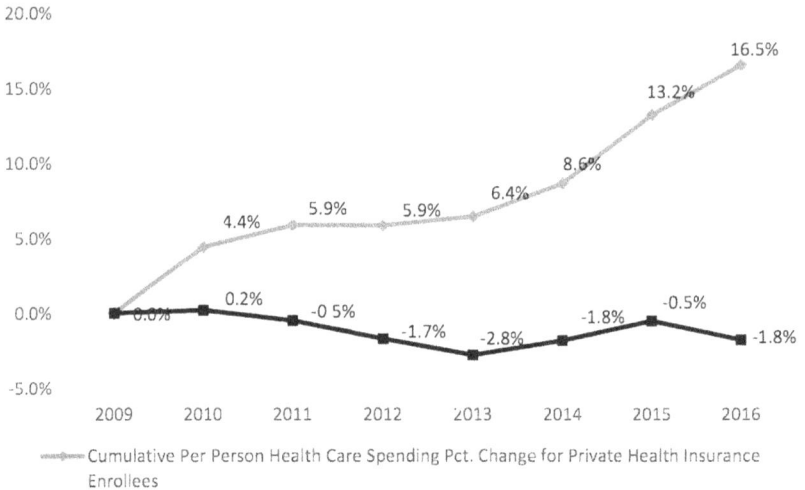

Source: National Health Expenditure Data –Historical, Centers for Medicare & Medicaid Services

to come to the realization that the private health insurance industry itself is a barrier to reform, and that it should be abandoned.

Dr. Michael Fine, family physician and author of the 2018 book, *Health Care Revolt: How to Organize, Build a Health Care System, and Resuscitate Democracy—All at the Same Time*, gives us this challenge:

Health care is for people, not for profit. We don't need more reform of the insurance market. Insurance and markets are problems, not the solution. We need a health care system that cares for every American in every community. [11]

FIGURE 12.3

AVERAGE STANDARDIZED PAYMENT RATES PER INPATIENT HOSPITAL STAY BY PRIMARY PAYER, 1996 - 2012

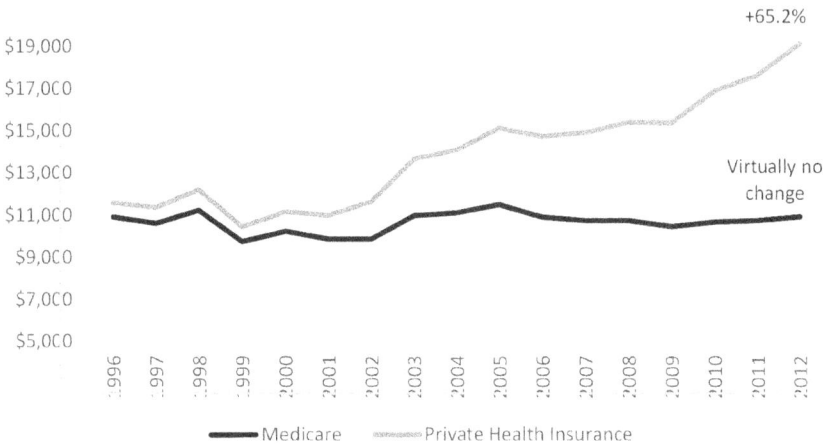

Source: 1996 - 2012 Medical Expenditure Panel Survey

Wendell Potter, adds this perspective from long experience as an executive with Cigna:

> *It's time for Democrats to stop proposing health care reform that relies on insurance companies to play fair. After two decades in the for-profit health insurance industry, I can assure you that they never will. They have no interest in doing anything that might in any way jeopardize profits. Their only interest is delivering profits to their shareholders. From that perspective, the status quo is very profitable. For everyone else, not so much. . . . Champion dramatic reforms, not half-measures.* [12]

4. Develop a national health profession workforce

plan with an increase in primary care.

All high-performing health care systems around the world have a strong foundation in primary care, which has these basic features:

1. First-contact care,
2. Longitudinal continuity over time,
3. Comprehensiveness, with capacity to manage majority of health problems, and
4. Coordination of care with other parts of the health care system. [13]

There is an extensive literature base over the years that primary care results in better health care for both individuals and populations in these four ways:

1. *Access is more available and efficient, with patients receiving more preventive services [14], having fewer preventable emergency room visits [15], and fewer hospitalizations [16]*

2. *Costs are better contained with strong primary care; knowing their patients well, primary care physicians order fewer tests than non-primary care specialists and can avoid unnecessary and inappropriate services by those specialists. [17]*

3. *Quality and outcomes of care are improved by primary care.* Earlier diagnosis and treatment result in better outcomes and lower mortality rates than for patients without a primary care base. [18,19]

4. *Primary care provides better coordination and integration of care.*

Non-primary care specialists are neither trained, oriented, nor equipped to recognize and manage the breadth of conditions common in primary care. Predictably, patients who see these specialists first for a new problem or chronic illness receive fragmented care through ping pong referrals to other specialists, resulting in higher costs and worse care. The Joint Commission on Accreditation of Healthcare Organizations has found that 80 percent of serious medical errors are associated with lack of communication or teamwork among specialists in hospitals. [20]

It is estimated that we will have a national shortage of up to 31,000 primary care physicians by 2025. [21] Family physicians are the mainstay of primary care in the U. S., since the great majority of general internists and pediatricians leave primary care for more highly reimbursed sub-specialties. Currently, less than 10 percent of U. S. medical school graduates enter family medicine residency programs. The vacuum in primary care has led to the proliferation of urgent care centers for first contact care, but without comprehensiveness, coordination, or continuity of care.

Despite the urgency of the primary care shortage, we still don't have a national physician workforce plan such as other countries with strong primary care have had for years. It is good news, however, that H. R. 1384 will establish an Office of Primary Care charged with increasing our primary care capacity.

5. Shift from a profit-driven business "ethic" to a service ethic for health care.

The prevailing norm in today's corporatized medical-industrial complex is to maximize revenues for CEOs and shareholders while squeezing employees, minimizing taxes, and leaving communities in the lurch when profits do not meet their expectations. National polls since the 1960s have shown a long descent in the public's trust and respect for corporations, especially pharmaceutical and private insurers, with only Congress and HMOs lower. [22, 23] NHI will change this dynamic toward a more service-oriented culture by implementing price and cost controls through bulk purchasing, negotiated global budgets, and other means.

6. Establish a non-partisan science-based National Institute, free from political influence, for ongoing evidence-based evaluation of treatments for efficacy and cost-effectiveness.

It should be a no-brainer that we have such an institute, especially since up to one-third of health care services provided in this country are inappropriate or unnecessary, with some even harmful. [24] Moreover, up to one-half of medical procedures provided each year by physicians are not supported by best scientific evidence. [25] Unfortunately, however, we still don't have such an institute after all these years. Evaluation of cost-effectiveness of treatments is even farther from political acceptance, remaining on the third rail of health care politics.

The ACA made a limited start toward a national body for evaluation of health care technology assessment by establishing the Patient-Centered Outcomes Research Institute (PCORI). However, it was not well funded and was restrained by this industry-friendly language in the ACA: "research findings may not be construed as mandates for practice guidelines, coverage recommendations, payment, or policy recommendations." [26] In addition, the ACA prohibited the use of cost-effectiveness or quality-adjusted life years (QALYs) in the Institute's recommendations. [27]

Here are some of the reasons that we still don't have an independent, well funded national body responsible for evaluating efficacy, quality and cost-effectiveness of medical treatments:

- Most medical research is biomedical and disease-oriented, with little emphasis on research oriented to primary care or health services.
- About two-thirds of drug research is funded by drug companies, conducted in for-profit commercial research networks with much less scientific rigor than studies by the National Institutes of Health (NIH).
- The FDA is beholden to the drug industry for the majority of its budget through user fees.
- Marketing efforts by drug companies are often disguised "science."
- There are many conflicts of interest in relationships between researchers, their institutions, and industry, with private gain often an issue over the public interest.
- A 2011 report found that 81 percent of physicians heading up panels writing clinical practice guidelines in cardiology had personal financial interests in companies affected by these guidelines. [28]
- Many studies with negative results are never reported, while many others that are published are written by for-profit ghost-writing agencies.

Past efforts to develop and maintain independent science-based federal agencies have met with political interference from industry over unfavorable reviews. The former Agency for Health Care Policy and Research (AHCPR), for example, had its funding cut and policy mission eliminated in the late 1990s when pressure was brought on Congress by spinal surgery providers and device manufacturers after release of AHCPR guidelines finding little evidence for the value of spinal fusion and favoring non-surgical approaches to low back pain. [29, 30]

There are good models of evidence-based institutes that evaluate health care services in other advanced countries around the world, especially the National Institute for Health and Clinical Excellence (NICE) in the United Kingdom. In 2008, Sir Michael Rawlins, the chairman of NICE, offered this advice to us:

> *The United States will one day have to take cost effectiveness into account. There is no doubt about it at all. You cannot keep on increasing your health care costs at the rate you are for so poor return. You are 29th in the world in life expectancy. You pay twice as much for health care as anyone else on God's earth.* [31]

The Political Battleground over Health Care Reform

Bipartisan support

There is broad and growing support among the public for Medicare for All (NHI). This support is even bipartisan, as shown by Figure 12.4. [32]

A recent comparison of all *Wall Street Journal/NBC* polls in 2010 and 2018 found a leftward shift by gender and all age groups. Democrats now consider themselves considerably more liberal than in 2010, as shown in Figure 12.5. This shift is also apparent in the 116th Congress, with 98 of the 235 House Democrats members of the Congressional Progressive Caucus. Moreover, 10 of the 16 announced Democratic presidential candidates have endorsed Bernie Sanders Medicare for All bill in the Senate. [33]

Jim Hightower reminds us, however, that the political spec-

FIGURE 12.4

Percentage of People Supporting Medicare for All, 2018

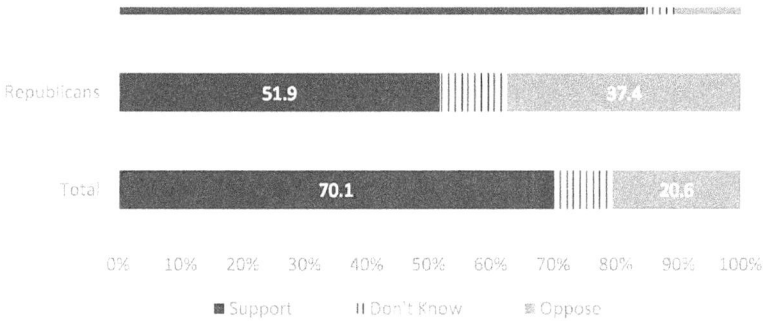

Source: Keller, M. Seventy Percent of Americans Support Medicare for All in New Poll, *The Hill*, August 23, 2018.

trum in this country is more than what many assume as mainly right to left:

> *The true political spectrum in America is not right to left, it's top to bottom. A bright progressive future awaits us if we join hands with the great progressive, racially inclusive majority of workaday people who're no longer in shouting distance for the economic and political elites at the top.* [34]

The 2018 mid-term elections were transformative. After the highest off-year turnout in a midterm election in 50 years, Democrats won the national congressional vote by a margin greater than that of the Tea Party Republicans in 2010 and women turned farther away from the Republican Party. Democrats gained almost 40 seats in the House, their largest pickup since the post-Watergate

FIGURE 12.5

Leftward Shift of Democrats By Gender and Age, 2010 to 2018

Percentage of Democrats that consider themselves:

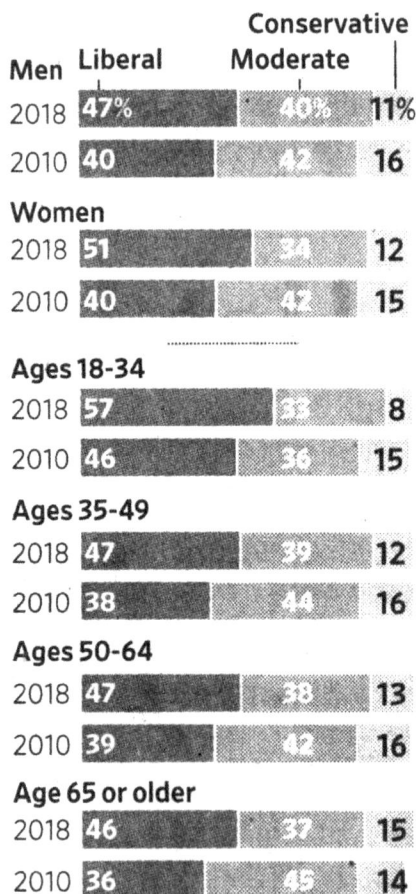

	Liberal	Moderate	Conservative
Men			
2018	47%	40%	11%
2010	40	42	16
Women			
2018	51	34	12
2010	40	42	15
Ages 18-34			
2018	57	33	8
2010	46	36	15
Ages 35-49			
2018	47	39	12
2010	38	44	16
Ages 50-64			
2018	47	38	13
2010	39	42	16
Age 65 or older			
2018	46	37	15
2010	36	45	14

Source: WSJ/NBC News Polls.

elections in 1974. The GOP lost badly in the House by running as an anti-immigrant party while the Democrats made big gains as a self-confident multicultural party. [35] The new House members include 33 women and 20 people of color. The new Congressional Progressive Caucus (CPC) is projected to include about 40 percent of House Democrats as the largest values-based caucus, with several members in House leadership positions. [36]

Medicare for All is a win-win for everybody, bringing access to essential health care wherever they live, with full choice of physician and hospital and no financial barriers to care. Their outcomes of care will improve through earlier diagnosis and treatment. Disparities of care will be removed as today's health care divide from one state to another is removed, and as individuals' incomes do not limit their access and quality of care. Physicians and other health professionals will welcome reduction of the bureaucracy of TrumpCare, with more time for direct patient care, higher practice satisfaction and less burnout. Employers will no longer be burdened by the increasing costs of covering their employees with health insurance as they gain a healthier workforce and the ability to better compete in a global market. Taxpayers will pay less than they do now for health care and insurance, as government at the state and federal level also save money.

Opposing forces

Despite a ground swell of public support for NHI, however, the vested interests are mounting a powerful coalition to defeat it, partly through heavy lobbying and a targeted disinformation campaign. Leading pharmaceutical, insurance and hospital lobbyists have formed The Partnership for America's Health Care Future, soon joined by the American Medical Association, to discredit Medicare for All. Eagan Kemp, health policy advocate with Public

Citizen, has suggested this more accurate name of this group as the Partnership for Profiting Off America's Health Care. [37]

Trump's demagoguery includes lies that NHI would "eviscerate Medicare, be a government takeover of health care, would ration care, patients would lose choice, doctors and hospitals would be put out of business, and there would be long waiting times to get care." [38] None of that would be true, of course, as access to care with more choice than exists today would become ensured by NHI. Meanwhile, a favorite and expected GOP attack line warns that Medicare for All would bring socialism, especially ironic since that was used as a boogie man to scare people away from Medicare when it was being debated in the early 1960s. [39]

Another approach being used by the opposition to Medicare for All is to play on the possible fears of patients losing their private health insurance. Some of these critics point out that some other countries with universal coverage have a limited role for private insurers. In Canada, for example, their single-payer system does not cover dental care or universal drug coverage. While both single-payer bills in Congress don't actually ban private health insurers, there would be no need for them, since our Medicare for All bills provide very comprehensive coverage without co-pays or deductibles. As Dr. Adam Gaffney, President of Physicians for a National Health Program, observes:

The only way to make room for a significant role for private insurance in the American context is to make the public system paltrier or skimpier, to impose onerous co-pays and deductibles, or to let the rich preferentially displace working-class people from hospital beds and doctors' offices. But it doesn't seem to make sense to punch holes in your own

*floor just to create work for a carpenter. That is particularly
true if your floor is your health care—and your carpenter is
an extractive insurance giant.* [40]

Need for wide public understanding

As the debate heats up in the new 116th Congress about how
to proceed on health care reform, there is increasing concern that
the public and legislators are confused and under-informed. A January 2019 Kaiser Health Tracking Poll found that large majorities
of respondents favored more incremental steps, such as a Medicare
buy-in plan for adults between ages 50 and 64 (77 percent) or a
Medicaid buy-in plan for individuals who don't receive coverage
through their employer (75 percent). [41] Meanwhile, 368 bipartisan
leaders in Congress signed on to support the private Medicare Advantage program, despite all of its problems discussed in earlier
chapters. [42]

Trump's proposed Medicare budget cut of $845 billion in
2020 seems certain to induce a complex and confusing debate
over Medicare itself. We can expect a broad public backlash to
any Medicare cuts, even by vested interests that oppose Medicare
for All. As one example, Chip Kahn, president and CEO of the
Federation of American Hospitals, has recently stated that: "Hospitals are less and less able to cover the cost of care for Medicare
patients; it is no time to gut Medicare." [43]

Trump's latest proposal is to say that a Texas lower court's
decision to rule the ACA unconstitutional, because of the compulsory individual mandate, should be sent up to the Supreme Court to
strike the entire law down. That decision's ruling will be reviewed
by the 5th District Court. If it is sent up to the Supreme Court, the
Department of Justice has already stated its agreement with the

lower court's decision. [44] In that event, Trump further claims that the Republicans will have a much better plan (an empty claim in the absence of any replacement plan even after eight plus years of trying!)

The Democrats, with strong control of the House, now have the best opportunity in many years to win Medicare for All. Trump's latest attempt to strike down the ACA will cede health care to the Democrats, and possibly even increase public support for Medicare for All. The Democrats, however, need to be united, not divided as they were in the run-up to the 2010 elections. They took an overly moderate pro-industry approach then, saying that "you can keep your insurance if you like it," and "we should build on the system's many strengths, not rebuild it entirely." They proposed the public option "to keep insurance honest," then gave up on that when corporate stakeholders won the day. All of that was a failed surrender-in-advance strategy, ending up with a narrow vote for the ACA in the House, passing there by a vote of just 219 to 212. [45]

Since the ACA has fallen so far short of urgently needed health care reform, Democrats in 2019 and 2020 need to learn from that experience. So far, internal debate within the Party is worrisome for its under informed centrist leanings weaken the Medicare for All Act of 2019 initiative put forward by real progressives. The center-left Center for American Progress, for example, is promoting its Medicare Extra for All, an expanded version of the public option that people could buy into. [46] Enactment of that or other incremental proposals would once again fail to provide universal coverage or resolve the nation's system problems of inadequate access to affordable health care.

Drs. Woolhandler and Himmelstein, whom we met in Chapter 9, published an important article in April 2019 that compares single-payer Medicare for All with four other incremental reform proposals being debated in Congress. They summarize these comparisons in this way:

The leading option for health reform in the United States would leave 36.2 million persons uninsured in 2027 while costs would balloon to nearly $6 trillion. [47] *That option is called the status quo. Other reasons why temporizing is a poor choice include the country's decreasing life expectancy, the widening mortality gap between the rich and the poor, and rising deductibles and drug prices. Even insured persons fear medical bills, commercial pressures permeate examination rooms, and physicians are burning out. In response to these health policy failures, many Democrats now advocate single-payer, Medicare-for-All reform, which until recently was a political nonstarter. Others are wary of frontally assaulting insurers and the pharmaceutical industry and advocate public-option plans or defending the Patient Protection and Affordable Care Act (ACA). Meanwhile, the Trump administration seeks to turbocharge market forces through deregulation and funneling more government funds through private insurers. Here, we highlight the probable effects of these proposals on how many persons would be covered, the comprehensiveness of coverage, and national health expenditures* (Table 12.2) [48]

There are other causes for concern. First, the ongoing efforts

TABLE 12.2

Characteristics of Major Health Reform Proposals, March, 2019

Characteristic	Medicare for All Single-Payer	Medicare for America
Chief sponsors	Jayapal (D-WA) and Sanders (I-VT)	DeLauro (D-CT) and Schakowsky (D-IL)
Provenance	Wagner-Murray-Dingell Bill (1948) Kennedy-Griffiths Bill (1970)	Javits Bill (1970) Center for American Progress (2018)
Enrollment	Automatic for all U.S. residents	Automatic for all U.S. residents unless an employer chooses to provide private coverage
Extent of coverage expansion	Universal	Universal
Comprehensiveness of coverage	Broad benefits; no copays or deductibles	Broad benefits; out-of-pocket costs capped at $3500
Role of private insurers	None	Large employers may choose to provide private insurance; MA continues with stricter regulations
Payment structure	Global budgets for hospitals; physicians paid according to a fee-for-service system or receive a salary; negotiated drug prices	Similar to the current Medicare system with increased primary care fees; negotiated drug prices
Funding mechanism	New taxes replace current out-of-pocket payments and premiums	New taxes; individual and employer premiums; out-of-pocket payments
Effect on overall national health expenditures	Initially similar to the status quo but lower thereafter because of administrative and drug savings	Probably moderate to large increases
Other major provisions	Coverage of long-term care varies	Premiums capped at 9.69% of income

Medicare Public Option	Medicaid Public Option	Trump White Paper and Budget Proposal
Merkley (D-OR) and Murphy (D-CT) Higgins (D-NY), Kaine (D-VA), and Bennet (D-CO) Schakowsky (D-IL) and Whitehouse (D-RI) Others	Schatz (D-HI) and Lujan (D-NM)	Executive branch actions and proposals; not yet in legislative form
Javits Bill (1962) Javits-Lindsay Bill (1964)	Lindsay proposal (1964)	Nixon proposals (1971) Long-Ribicoff Bill (1973) Medicare Modernization Act (2003)
Available as an option on ACA exchanges	States may choose to provide this strategy as an option on ACA exchanges	Little change
Modest	Very modest; some states would probably decline to participate	Coverage would probably decrease
Somewhat broader than the current Medicare plan; out-of-pocket costs are similar to or somewhat lower than those under current ACA plans	Similar to ACA exchange plans; states set copays and deductibles	Weakens ACA mandates on coverage of "essential benefits" and preexisting conditions; relaxes network-adequacy standards; encourages higher deductibles
Probably modestly reduced	Probably modestly reduced	Private MA plans expand at the expense of traditional Medicare
Little change	Medicaid adopts Medicare payment rates	Accelerated shift from a fee-for-service system to value-based purchasing and ACOs
Enrollee-paid premiums	Enrollee-paid premiums	Proposed cuts of $1.5 trillion to Medicaid and $818 billion to Medicare over 10 y
Small increases	Small increases	Uncertain
Some proposals increase ACA subsidies	Premiums capped at 9.5% of income	Lifts moratorium on new for-profit specialty hospitals; expands the scope of practice of nonphysician providers; relaxes standards for FMGs; overrides states' "any-willing-provider" and certificate-of-need regulations

Source: Woolhandler, S, Himmelstein, DU. Medicare for All and its rivals: new offshoots of old health policy roots. Ideas and Opinions. *Ann Intern Med*, April; 2, 2019.

of the Democratic Congressional Campaign Committee (DCCC) to warn candidates in the 2018 and 2020 campaigns about the political liabilities of their endorsing single-payer Medicare for All, fearing attacks from Republicans for favoring "socialized medicine." [49] And second, establishment Democratic leaders in the House are rolling out their incremental bill to protect the ACA from Trump's sabotage, but not support H. R. 1384 Improved and Expanded Medicare for All. [50]

As Dr. Don McCanne, former president of Physicians for a National Health Program, observes:

> *I'm much more worried about our friends than our enemies. A decade ago our friends kicked us out of the negotiations and brought us Obamacare. By now we could have had everyone covered at a cost we could afford, but instead we have tens of millions uninsured and underinsured who are losing their choices in health care while our national health care expenditures increase at twice the rate of inflation, all the while perpetuating suffering, hardship, and premature death.* [51]

The question among Democratic hopefuls in the 2020 presidential campaigns is whether support for Medicare for All should be a litmus test for their candidacies. Some are already backing away to a more incremental non-universal coverage approach, but Kamala Harris has bravely put her support for Medicare for All right out the gate at a CNN town hall:

> *Government should eliminate private health insurance and fund virtually all health care services directly. The idea*

is that everyone gets access to medical care and you don't have to go through the process of going through an insurance company, having them give you approval, going through the paperwork, all of the delay that may require. Let's eliminate all of that. Let's move on." [52]

Bonne Castillo, RN, executive director of National Nurses United, responds to the corporate and GOP attacks on Medicare for All this way:

We expect corporate attacks. But the people see through them. We expect our future leaders to see through them, too. Every other modern nation on earth has proven to us that guaranteed health care is possible. So we'll be watching closely to see which presidential candidates support Medicare for All, and which candidates fall short, by backing half measures. . . When it comes to those seeking the highest office in the land, the people's vote hinges on a critical question: Whose side are you on? [53]

Conclusion

Incremental change on health care, in the midst of a heated battle between corporate stakeholders in the status quo and those pushing for real reform, is a trap that comes up every time. The outcome of the battle on this occasion will depend on political will and unity among Democrats, which already shows signs of fraying. Based on today's crisis in U. S. health care, we really need to act in the public interest this time, not fold as occurred in 2010 with the ACA. As Martin Luther King, Jr. said in 1964: "the time is always ripe to do right." [54]

Public Citizen observes the timeliness of the Medicare for All movement today in this way:

We are at a rare moment in time, in the window of what might be a once-in-a-century opportunity to boldly reshape our health care system to expand and improve access to care such that we could potentially leap-frog the countries that currently outperform us in health outcomes. Such a clear surge in support for Medicare for All that our nation is experiencing holds the promise of taking us from worst-to-first when it comes to providing guaranteed access to health care. [55]

As all the powerful forces for and against this kind of reform collide, we all need to ask ourselves whose side we're on, and answer for the common good. As this plays out, the wisdom of Mahatma Gandhi is reassuring:

First they ignore you, then they laugh at you, then they fight you, then you win.

References

1. Flavelle, C. Obamacare's dropout are middle-age men. *Bloomberg News*, March 17, 2014.
2. Higginbotham, T. Medicare for All is even better than you thought. *Jacobin*, December 3, 2018.
3. Krugman, P. The world of U. S. health care economics is downright scary. *Seattle Post-Intelligencer*, September 26, 2006: B1.
4. Himmelstein, DU, Woolhandler, S. The post-launch problem: The Affordable Care Act's persistently high administrative costs. *Health Affairs Blog*, May 27, 2015.
5. Herman, B. Medicaid's unmanaged managed care. *Modern Healthcare*, April 30, 2016.
6. Frakt, A. *Private Vs. Public Prices. Academy Health Blog*, January 13, 2017.

7. *National Health Expenditure Data—Historical.* Centers for Medicare and Medicaid Services.

8. Ockerman, E. It costs $685 billion a year to subsidize U. S. health insurance. *Bloomberg News,* May 23, 2018.

9. Fine, M. *Health Care Revolt: How to Organize, Build a Health Care System, and Resuscitate Democracy—All at the Same Time.* Oakland, CA. *PM Press,* 2018, p. 138.

10. Potter, W. Take it from me, tweaks won't fix health care. Democrats should focus on Medicare for All. *USA Today,* December 14, 2018.

11. Starfield, B. Is primary care essential? *The Lancet* 344 (8930): 1129-1133, 1994.

12. Bindman, AB, Grumbach, K, Osmond, D et al. Primary care receipt of preventive services. *J Gen Intern Med* 11: 269-276, 1996.

13. Hurley, RE, Freund, DA, Taylor, DE. Emergency room use and primary care case management: evidence from four Medicaid demonstration programs. *Am J Pub Health 79*: 843-846, 1988.

14. Parchman, ML, Culler, S. Primary care physicians and avoidable hospitalization. *J Fam Pract* 39: 122-128, 1994.

15. Greenfield, S, Nelson, EC, Zubkoff, M et al. Variations in resource utilization among medical specialties and systems of care: Results from the Medical Outcomes Study. *JAMA* 267 (12): 1624-1630, 1992.

16. Ferrante, Gonzales, EC, Pal, N et al. Effects of physician supply on early detection of breast cancer. *J Am Board of Fam Pract* 13: 408-414, 2000.

17. Franks, P, Fiscella, K. Primary care physicians and specialists as personal physicians: health care expenditures and mortality experience. *J Fam Pract* 47: 103-104, 1998.

18. Health blog. Joint Commission-Hospital Collaboration targets hand-offs. *Wall Street Journal,* October 21, 2010.

19. Press release. Association of American Medical Colleges (AAMC). March 3, 2015.

20. Pearlstein, S. When shareholder capitalism comes to town. *The American Prospect,* March/April 2014: 40-48.

21. Harris poll on profits and ethics in health care. *The Harris Poll.* January 17, 2017.

22. Caper, P. The ills of money-driven medicine. Op-Ed. *Bangor Daily News,* May 21, 2012.

23. Patashnik, E. Why American doctors keep doing expensive procedures that don't work. *VOX*, February 14 2018.

24. Gerber, AS, Patashnik, EM, Doherty, D et al. The public wants information, not board mandates, from comparative effectiveness research. *Health Affairs* 29 (10): 1879, 2010.

25. AAMC Government Relations. *Summary of Patient-Centered Outcomes Research Provisions*, March 2010.

26. Mendelson, TB, Melzer, M, Campbell, EG et al. Conflicts of interest in cardiovascular clinical practice guidelines. *Arch Intern Med* 171 (6): 577-584, 2011.

27. Deyo, RA, Psaty, BM, Simon, G et al. The messenger under attack: Intimidation of researchers by special interest groups. *N Engl J Med* 336: 1176, 1997.

28. Deyo, RA, Nachemson, A, Mirza, SK. Spinal-fusion surgery—the case for restraint. *N Eng. J Med* 350: 722-726, 2004.

29. Rawlins, M. As quoted by Silberman, J. Britain weighs the social cost of high-priced drugs. *NPR*, July 3, 2008.

30. *Public Citizen. The Case for Medicare-For-All*, Washington, D. C., February 4, 2019, p. 36.

31. Pollin, R, Heintz, J, Arno, P et al. *In-Depth Analysis by Team of UMass Amherst Economists Shows Viability of Medicare for All*. Amherst, MA, November 30, 2018.

32. Keller, M. Seventy Percent of Americans Support 'Medicare for All' in New Poll, *The Hill*, August 23, 2018.

33. Epstein, RJ, Thomas, K. Democratic candidates split over Party's leftward drift. *Wall Street Journal*, March 21, 2019: A 1.

34. Hightower, J. *The Hightower Lowdown*, August 2018.

35. Greenberg, SB. Trump is beginning to lose his grip. *New York Times*, November 17, 2018.

36. Viebeck, E, Kane, P. 'They're not asking permission to do things': Democrats brace for robust freshman class. *The Washington Post*, December 31, 2018.

37. Fang, L, Surgey, N. Lobbyist documents reveal health care industry battle plan against Medicare for All. *The Intercept*, November 20, 2018.

38. Trump, DJ. Donald Trump: Democrats' Medicare for All plan will demolish promises to seniors. *USA Today*, October 10, 2018.

39. Itkowitz, C. GOP argument against 'Medicare for All' doesn't make sense. *The Washington Post*, September 10, 2018.

40. Gaffney, A. We don't need private health insurance. New single-payer plans don't need to worry about carving out roles for health-care profiteers. *The Nation*, February 18, 2019.

41. Kirzinger, A, Munana, C, Brodie, M. KFF Health Tracking Poll—January 2019: The public on next steps for the ACA and proposals to expand coverage. *Kaiser Family Foundation*, January 23, 2019.

42. AHIP thanks Congress for the overwhelming support for Medicare Advantage. *America's Health Insurance Plans* (AHIP), February 7, 2019.

43. Olorunnipa, T, Sullivan, S. Proposed Medicare cuts may become issue in 2020 race. *The Washington Post*, March 13, 2019.

44. Schwarz, C. Department of Justice states support for total invalidation of the Affordable Care Act. Medicare Rights Center, March 28, 2019.

45. Geyman, JP. Crisis in U. S. health care: Corporate power still blocks reform. *Intl J Health Services* on line, October 3, 2017, p. 4.

46. Grim, R. The special interests behind Rep. Pramila Jayapal's Medicare for All are not the usual suspects. *The Intercept*, February 27, 2019.

47. Sisko, AM, Keehan, SP, Poisal, JA et al. National health expenditure projections, 2018-2017: economic and demographic trends drive spending and enrollment growth. *Health Affairs* (Millwood), 2019, 38:10, 377.

48. Woolhandler, S, Himmelstein, DU. Medicare for All and its rivals: new offshoots of old health policy roots. Ideas and Opinions. *Ann Intern Med*, April; 2, 2019.

49. Habercorn, J. The 2 words you can't say in a Democratic ad. *Politico*, June 8, 2018.

50. Pear, R. House Democrats to unveil plan to expand health coverage. *New York Times*, March 25, 2019.

51. McCanne, D. Let's get it right: Medicare for All is a huge bargain. *Quote of the Day*, August 13, 2018.

52. Brownstein, R. The coming Democratic drama over Medicare for All. *The Atlantic*, January 31, 2019.

53. Castillo, B. 2020 candidates will have to choose a side—the health insurance industry or the people. *Common Dreams*, February 7, 2019.

54. King ML, Jr. City Temple, London, England, December 7, 1964.

55. Ibid # 30, p. 8.

GLOSSARY

Accountable care organization (ACO): These are loosely designed managed care organizations involving hospital systems, physicians, and insurers, established under the ACA in an effort to contain health care costs. They are expected to provide care for a population of at least 5,000 people for a period of at least three years, with the goal to improve coordination and quality of care in and out of the hospital.

Actuarial value: The percentage of total average health care costs that a health plan will pay for covered services. The ACA set up four "metal" levels of health plans through the exchanges—ranging from bronze, which covers only 60 percent of costs, to platinum, which covers 90 percent of costs.

Adverse selection: This occurs when lower-risk individuals are split off by insurers from a larger risk pool in order to minimize their financial risk and increase their profits. The smaller risk pool of higher-risk individuals that results requires higher costs of treatment. Adverse selection is the Achilles' heel of capitation, since for-profit HMOs and some physicians are often tempted to selectively care for healthier patients while avoiding the care of sicker patients.

America's Health Insurance Plans (AHIP): This is the insurance industry's national trade group representing about 1,300 private insurance companies. It was formed in 2003 by the merger of the American Association of Health Plans (AAHP) and the Health Insurance Association of America (HIAA).

Capitation: A method of payment for patient care services used by managed care organizations, such as health maintenance organizations (HMOs), to reimburse providers under contractual agreements. Payment rates are set in advance, and are paid monthly or annually regardless of what services are actually provided to covered patients.

Consumer Directed Health Care (CDHC): A strategy intended to contain health care costs by shifting more responsibility to consumers in choosing and paying for their own health care. This theory of cost-containment has been supported by many economists and most conservatives for years, but has failed as a cost-containment measure while leading many lower-income patients to delay or forgo necessary care.

Co-insurance: This refers to the percentage of health care costs which are not covered by insurance and which the individual must pay. Many insurance plans cover 80 percent of the costs of hospital and physician care, leaving 20 percent to be paid by patients or by supplemental insurance.

Community rating: A method for setting premiums for health insurance based on the average cost of health care for the covered population in a geographic area. This method shares risk across all covered individuals, whether sick or well, so that the healthy help to subsidize care of the sick who otherwise may not be able to afford coverage on their own. Community rating was abandoned by most private health insurers after the 1960s, as experience rating spread throughout the industry.

Cost effectiveness: When applied to health care, cost-effectiveness attempts to estimate the value for expenditures on procedures or services that is returned to patients, such as longer life, better quality of life, or both. Cost-effectiveness analysis (CEA) is the scientific technique used to measure costs and efficacy of alternative treatments in order to estimate their economic value, which then are typically measured in quality-adjusted life years (QALYs).

Co-payment: Flat fee charged directly to patients whenever they seek health care services or drug prescriptions regardless of their insurance coverage. In today's environment, co-payments are increasing across the health care marketplace to the point of being a financial barrier to care for many lower-income people.

Cost-sharing: This refers to requirements that patients pay directly out-of-pocket for some portion of their health care costs. The level of cost-sharing varies considerably from one health plan to another, and for many people is another financial barrier to access to necessary health care.

Death spiral: This term describes the progressive effects of adverse selection in shrinking a risk pool into a smaller population of high-risk individuals requiring expensive care. As a result of "cherry picking" by for-profit health insurers, public programs such as traditional Medicare are placed at risk because of reduced cross subsidies from the healthy to the sick.

Deductible: Out-of-pocket costs which patients must pay before their insurance coverage kicks in for subsequent costs. This amount is required to be met each year. The trend today is toward plans with high deductibles, some up to $10,000 or more, constituting yet another financial barrier to care.

Defined benefits: This term is applied when an insurance plan offers a pre-determined set of benefits to all enrollees. Traditional Medicare is such an example, with covered benefits authorized by law.

Defined contributions: This is the polar opposite from defined benefits. In this instance, a fixed set of benefits is not provided by the insurer, whether public or private. Instead a defined contribution is made toward the costs of coverage, such as by an employer or a privatized public plan. See also Premium Support and Vouchers.

The Emergency Medical Treatment and Active Labor Act (EMTALA): This was enacted by Congress in 1986 in order to ensure public access to emergency services regardless of ability to pay. Medicare-participating hospitals that offer emergency services are required to provide stabilizing treatment for all emergency medical conditions, including active labor.

Employer mandate: A policy that requires all or most employers to provide health insurance for their employees. The Affordable Care Act includes this approach, but allows some exceptions to this requirement, which has also been delayed for a year.

Employer sponsored insurance (ESI): A voluntary system established during the wartime economy of the 1940s whereby many employers provide health insurance coverage to their employees. This system has been gradually unraveling for years, now covering less than two-thirds of the non-elderly workforce, with many employers covering less through defined contribution and high-deductible plans.

Employee Retirement Income Security Act of 1974 (ERISA): Enacted in 1974 before the advent of managed care, ERISA was originally intended to protect pension plans, but soon became a loophole in states' attempts to regulate abuses by private health insurers. Under ERISA, all self-funded health plans are exempt from state regulations, as are many managed care organizations. ERISA does not apply to Medicare, Medicaid, and insurance provided by government employers.

Experience rating: This is the current norm in private U.S. health insurance markets, as opposed to the community rating tradition originally established by Blue Cross in the 1930s. Under experience rating, insurers avoid high-risk individuals and groups and increase premiums based upon illnesses experienced by enrollees. Experience rating weakens the ability of health insurance to share risk across a large risk pool of healthy and sick individuals.

Favorable risk selection: This is the process by which insurers screen potential enrollees according to health status, avoiding higher-risk sick individuals and groups in favor of healthier enrollees requiring less costly care—the opposite of adverse selection.

Federal poverty level (FPL): Annual income levels updated annually by the federal government defining poverty levels based on size of household. These are the guidelines for FFY 2019:

Family Size	100%	133%	200%
1	$12,490	$16,612	$24,980
2	$16.910	$22,490	$33,820
3	$21,330	$28,369	$42,660
4	$25,750	$34,248	$51,500

Fee-for-service (FFS): A common method of reimbursement for health services provided, such as by visit procedure, laboratory test or imaging study. Fees are often based on a fixed fee schedule or on more complex relative value scales. See also Resource-Based Relative Value Scale.

Fiscal Intermediary: Private insurers that have contracted with Medicare since the mid-1960s to administer hospitalization insurance under Part A of Medicare. Blue Cross has held most of these contracts over the years. In this capacity, insurers are empowered to make coverage and reimbursement decisions and to provide related administrative services

Formulary: Lists of drugs updated at regular intervals which can be prescribed by physicians for enrollees in specific health plans. Formulary development is a contentious area, with the pharmaceutical industry arguing for wider coverage lists while health plans strive to balance cost, efficacy, and safety issues against patients' access to medically necessary medications.

Gross domestic product (GDP): An economic indicator that measures the total output of everything produced by all the people and companies in a given country from year to year.

Guaranteed issue: This is typically opposed by the private health insurance industry because of the likelihood of adverse selection. The Affordable Care Act gives consumers new protections by banning insurers from denial of coverage because of pre-existing conditions.

Global budgets: These are annual negotiated costs under single-payer national health insurance that will cover all costs of a hospital or other health care facility on an annual global basis.

Health exchanges: These were established under the ACA, for participating states or the federal government to provide a marketplace where consumers can shop for health plans that meet their pocket book and needs.

Health maintenance organization (HMO): HMOs are organizations that provide a broad range of services, coordinated by primary care physicians on a prepaid basis for enrollees. The earliest HMOs were established in the 1940s and 1950s, such as Kaiser Permanente and Group Health Cooperative of Puget Sound. They are integrated systems where physicians are salaried and work only with that HMO. Later years have seen the emergence of mostly for-profit HMOs that are looser structures contracting with physicians in independent practices who agree to provide managed care on a capitation basis for a panel of patients.

Health savings account (HSA): These were authorized under the Medicare Prescription Drug, Improvement, and Modernization Act of 2003 (MMA) as part of an effort to contain health care costs by shifting more financial responsibility to consumers for their health care choices and decisions. Employer and employee contributions to an HSA are tax-free when accompanied by high-deductible insurance policies. While providing new investment opportunities for healthy individuals, HSAs provide little financial protection against the costs of serious illness.

High-deductible health insurance plans (HDHI): There has been a growing trend in recent years for insurers and employers to offer HDHI plans with high cost-sharing requirements and annual deductibles as high as $10,000. These policies are typically associated with health savings accounts and provide little coverage or security for people experiencing significant medical expenses.

High-risk pool: With the goal to help people who have been denied coverage in the individual market, high-risk pools have been established by many states with federal and state funding as a means of pooling risk with others facing the same problem. The Affordable Care Act provides additional support for these high-risk pools, but their experience has been mostly disappointing because of the costs involved.

Individual market: The individual market is much smaller than that of employer-sponsored insurance. Many people with significant health issues find it difficult to gain affordable coverage in the individual market. The Affordable Care Act helps to a certain degree, especially by eliminating insurers' denial of coverage because of pre-existing conditions and providing subsidies for eligible enrollees, but coverage remains unaffordable for some.

Limited benefit plan: These are policies being marketed by private insurers to employers and healthier people with restricted benefits and annual caps as low as $1,000 to $2,500.

Managed care: Although this term has often become ambiguous and unclear in common usage, it expresses a relatively new relationship between purchasers, insurers, and providers of care. To a variable extent, organizations that pay for patient care have also taken on the role of making decisions about patient care management. In practice, however, "managed care" is often more managed reimbursement than care, with the possibility of perverse financial incentives to skimp on necessary services. There are three basic types of managed care organizations— preferred provider organizations (PPOs), group and staff model HMOs, and independent practice associations (IPA) HMOs.

Medicaid: This is a federal-state health insurance program, enacted in 1965, that covers low-income people who meet variable and changing state eligibility requirements. Most elderly, disabled, and blind individuals who receive assistance through the federal Supplemental Security Income (SSI) program are covered under Medicaid, which is also the main payer of nursing home costs. Current budget deficits in federal and state budgets threaten this vital safety net program, which provides last-resort coverage for about one in six Americans, including one-fifth of all children in the U.S.

Medicaid coverage gap: This refers to the approximately five million people who would have qualified for expanded Medicaid under the ACA but who live in states that opted out of Medicaid expansion. They are lower-income, uninsured adults with incomes above Medicaid eligibility levels but below the federal poverty level, so that they cannot qualify for either Medicaid or subsidies through the health exchanges.

Medical loss ratio (MLR): The medical loss ratio is that part of the premium dollar spent by insurers on direct medical care. Private insurers typically try to keep their MLR below the 80 or 85 percent level required by the Affordable Care Act, but have found ways to game that requirement by including other non-patient care expenses under "direct medical care."

Medical necessity: An elusive but important term which is applied to treatments and health care services that can be judged on the basis of clinical evidence to be effective and indicated as essential medical care. It is an ongoing challenge for health professionals, insurers, payers and policymakers to define medical necessity as part of coverage policy, made more difficult as costs are considered and as new treatments are brought into use.

Medical underwriting: This is the process used by health insurers to calculate higher premiums to be charged to individual or group applicants at higher risk of illness. Medical underwriting was considered unethical in the early years of private health insurance in this country, but became the industry norm after the 1960s and is typically based on annual review of claims experience. Although the ACA prohibits insurers from denying coverage based on pre-existing conditions, private insurers still have other ways to avoid higher-risk enrollees, such as by selective marketing and tiering of benefits.

Medicare: A federal health insurance program for the elderly and disabled enacted in 1965 that now covers about 54 million Americans age 65 and older as well as younger adults with permanent disabilities, including those with chronic kidney failure. Traditional (Original) Medicare covers about one-half of beneficiaries' health care expenses, and accounts for about one-fifth of personal national health expenditures. There are four components of Medicare today:

Part A: Hospitalization insurance
Part B: Supplementary medical insurance
Part C: Private Medicare plans, now Medicare Advantage
Part D: Prescription drug coverage, starting in 2006.

Medicare Advantage: Private health plans authorized by Medicare legislation in 2003 as the sequel to Medicare + Choice programs. Most are HMOs, though many are preferred provider organizations (PPOs).

Medigap: These are private supplemental plans, available to people that already have Medicare Parts A and B, that help to cover some costs that Medicare does not cover, such as co-payments, coinsurance and deductibles. Medigap policies generally do not cover vision or dental care, hearing aids, eyeglasses or private duty nursing.

Monopsony purchasing: Purchasing of goods and services by a single buyer, such as bulk purchasing of prescription drugs by the Veterans Administration using the leverage of its population to obtain discounted prices from drug manufacturers.

National health insurance (NHI): A national health insurance program that would provide universal coverage to the entire U.S. population for necessary health care. It would be a single-payer system, government-financed with a private delivery system. Through simplified administration, it would provide more efficiency and cost containment than the current multi-payer market-based system while offering new opportunities to improve accountability and quality assurance within the system.

Network providers and hospitals: This designation is used by ACOs, HMOs and PPOs to indicate providers within networks of providers and hospitals. Networks today are typically set up by insurers and ACOs as ways to reduce their costs, not to improve continuity or quality of patient care. Patients are often penalized by having to pay more outside of these networks in order to receive care by their physicians and hospitals of choice.

Overpayments: These are administratively set payments to Medicare Advantage plans in excess of fee-for-service payments under traditional Medicare. Since the early years of private Medicare plans, insurers have successfully entrenched the concept that they should be paid more by the federal government than traditional Medicare, leading more to their increased profits than service to patients.

Pay for performance (P4P): An umbrella term referring to various approaches intended to improve the quality, efficiency and value of health care. A number of Medicare demonstration projects have been carried out over the last ten years to test this concept, which has been incorporated into the ACA. So far, P4P initiatives have not been found to contain costs or improve the quality of care.

Pre-existing condition: In the process of medical underwriting as insurers evaluate applicants for coverage, medical conditions which pre-date the application are scrutinized as they relate to future health risks. In the past, they have been used by insurers to deny coverage or raise initial premiums if coverage is offered. This practice has been eliminated by the ACA.

Preferred provider organization (PPO): A kind of health plan wherein providers agree to accept set discounted fees in exchange for the practice-building opportunity of being listed as a "preferred provider." Many patients favor a PPO that includes their physicians to an arbitrary network that excludes their chosen providers.

Premium support: This is a strategy promoted by its supporters intended to limit the government's financial responsibility to Medicare beneficiaries by shifting from a defined benefit program to a defined contribution approach. Under premium support, the government would pay a set amount toward the cost of a plan, whether FFS. HMO, or PPO, with enrollees responsible for any price differences. See also voucher.

Quality assurance: A broad field that has developed over the years with the goal to improve the quality of clinical practice, reduce the rate of medical errors, and improve patient care outcomes. This is an ongoing and difficult challenge, with evidence-based clinical practice guidelines an integral part of the process.

Risk adjustment: A complex technical process intended to estimate the difference in health status and risk in populations enrolled in Medicare private plans compared to fee for service (FFS) Medicare. It is well documented that private plans attract healthier patients requiring less costly care than traditional Medicare through favorable risk selection. Risk adjustment techniques so far have been too crude to deal with this problem.

Risk pool: A group of people considered together in order to price their insurance coverage. The larger and more diverse the group in terms of health status, the more effective insurance can be in having healthier individuals share the higher costs of care of sicker individuals while assuring the most affordable insurance premiums for the entire group.

Single-payer: A single national financing system that covers an entire population. Traditional Medicare in the U. S. is one example, as is the Veterans Administration for veterans' health care. The U. S. has had legislation put forward in Congress on a number of occasions, such as H.R. 1384 today, that would enact such a system of universal health insurance for all U. S. residents. But so far there has not been the political will to overcome the resistance of private corporate stakeholders in our current market-based system.

Socialized medicine: Socialized medicine refers to a publicly-financed government owned and operated health care delivery system. The National Health Service in England is one such example, with government ownership of hospitals and physicians as salaried employees. The V.A. in this country is another example. National health insurance, as an expanded and improved Medicare for All program coupled with a private delivery system, would in no way be socialized medicine.

Social insurance: Social insurance is compulsory, usually provided by a public agency, and spreads the financial risk of illness across an entire population, making its costs affordable to a large population. This in marked contrast to private insurance, which is voluntary, provided by private insurers (usually for-profit) which selectively enroll better risks, thereby making coverage unaffordable or otherwise unavailable to higher-risk individuals. Traditional Medicare has been a social insurance program over the last 54 years, but is threatened by further privatization.

Underinsurance: As the costs of health care continue to rise at rates several times the cost-of-living and median family incomes, fewer people can afford insurance with comprehensive benefits. It they can afford coverage at all, they find themselves challenged by high levels of cost-sharing. The Commonwealth Fund has defined underinsurance on the basis of the proportion of total family income spent on health care (i.e. more than 10 percent of income, more that 5 percent of income if below 200 percent of federal poverty level, or deductibles equal to or exceeding 5 percent of income).

Universal coverage: This term describes countries that provide health insurance to all citizens regardless of age, income, or health status. The U.S. is an outlier among advanced countries around the world in not having universal coverage while spending far more than any other country for health care.

Utilization management (UM): A cost containment strategy used by Medicare, Medicaid, and many private plans that monitors the clinical activities of physicians. Payments for some services are denied if considered by the payer to be unnecessary. Critics of this approach contend that UM is an unwarranted intrusion into the physician-patient relationship, involves a burdensome administrative hassle for caregivers, and doesn't save much money anyway.

Voucher: A grant of money for a specific purpose, such as for meals or transportation. Conservatives have promoted the idea of vouchers for years as a way to reduce the government's responsibility for Medicare costs. Vouchers would shift Medicare from a program with defined benefits to one of defined contributions by the government to Medicare beneficiaries. Critics see this approach as a threat to the integrity and viability of the Medicare program, by also opening the door to stepwise further reductions in the level of government funding.

A

J

K

O

P

Q

R

S

ABOUT THE AUTHOR

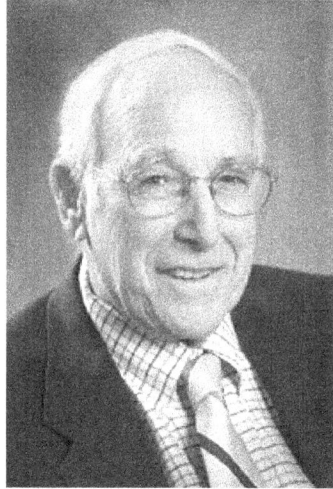

John Geyman, M.D. is professor emeritus of family medicine at the University of Washington School of Medicine in Seattle, where he served as Chairman of the Department of Family Medicine from 1976 to 1990. As a family physician with over 21 years in academic medicine, he also practiced in rural communities for 13 years. He was the founding editor of *The Journal of Family Practice* (1973 to 1990) and the editor of *The Journal of the American Board of Family Medicine* from 1990 to 2003. Since 1990 he has been involved with research and writing on health policy and health care reform.

His most recent book was *TrumpCare: Lies, Broken Promises, How It Is Failing, and What Should Be Done?* (2018). Earlier books include: *Crisis in U.S. Health Care: Corporate Power vs. the Common Good* (2017), *The Human Face of ObamaCare: Promises vs. Reality and What Comes Next* (2016), *How Obamacare Is Unsustainable: Why We Need a Single-Payer Solution For All Americans* (2015), *Health Care Wars: How Market Ideology and Corporate Power Are Killing Americans* (2012), *Souls On a Walk: An Enduring Love Story Unbroken by Alzheimer's* (2012),

Breaking Point: How the Primary Care Crisis Threatens the Lives of Americans (2011), *Hijacked: The Road to Single Payer in the Aftermath of Stolen Health Care Reform (2010), The Cancer Generation: Baby Boomers Facing a Perfect Storm* (2009), *Do Not Resuscitate: Why the Health Insurance Industry Is Dying (2008), The Corrosion of Medicine: Can the Profession Reclaim Its Moral Legacy* (2008), *Shredding the Social Contract: The Privatization of Medicare* (2006), *Falling Through the Safety Net: Americans Without Health Insurance (2005), The Corporate Transformation of Health Care: Can the Public Interest Still Be Served? (2004),* and *Health Care in America: Can Our Ailing System Be Healed?* (2002), and *The Modern Family Doctor and Changing Medical Practice* (1971).

John has also published two pamphlets following the approach of Thomas Paine in 1775-1776: *Common Sense About Health Care Reform in America* (2017), and *Common Sense: U.S. Health Care at a Crossroads in the 2018 Congress.*

He also served as the president of Physicians for a National Health Program from 2005 to 2007, and is a member of the National Academy of Medicine.